IRRITABLE BOWEL SYNDROME

First published in French in 2016 by Les Publications Modus Vivendi Inc. under the title
Syndrome du côlon irritable.
© Alexandra Leduc and Les Publications Modus Vivendi Inc., 2016

MODUS VIVENDI PUBLISHING
55 Jean-Talon Street West
Montreal, Quebec H2R 2W8
CANADA

modusvivendipublishing.com

Publisher: Marc G. Alain
Editorial director: Isabelle Jodoin
Content and copy editor: Nolwenn Gouezel
Translator: Donna Vekteris
English-language editor: Carol Sherman
English-language copy editor: Maeve Haldane
Graphic designers: Émilie Houle and Gabrielle Lecomte
Page layout: Hélène Lamoureux
Food and author's photographer: André Noël (anoelphoto.com)
Food stylist: Gabrielle Dalessandro
Additional photography:
Pages 6, 8, 13, 14, 21, 23, 27, 28, 29, 31, 33, 37, 38, 39, 40, 41, 42, 43, 44, 45, 46, 47, 48, 49, 50, 51, 52, 53, 54, 55, 56, 57, 60, 62, 66, 77, 78, 87, 105, 108, 110, 122, 130: Dreamstime.com
Pages 17, 37, 49, 56, 84, 133: iStock
Page 134: Camille Gyrya (camillegyrya.com)

ISBN: 978-1-77286-038-2 (PAPERBACK)

ISBN: 978-1-77286-039-9 (PDF)
ISBN: 978-1-77286-040-5 (EPUB)
ISBN: 978-1-77286-041-2 (KINDLE)

Legal deposit — Bibliothèque and Archives nationales du Québec, 2016
Legal deposit — Library and Archives Canada, 2016

We gratefully acknowledge the financial support of the Government of Canada through the Canada Book Fund (CBF) for our publishing activities.

Government of Quebec — Tax Credit for Book Publishing — Program administered by SODEC

Printed in Canada

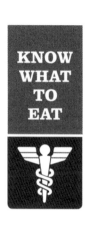

IRRITABLE BOWEL SYNDROME

21 DAYS OF MENUS

Alexandra Leduc, RD

MODUS VIVENDI

CONTENTS

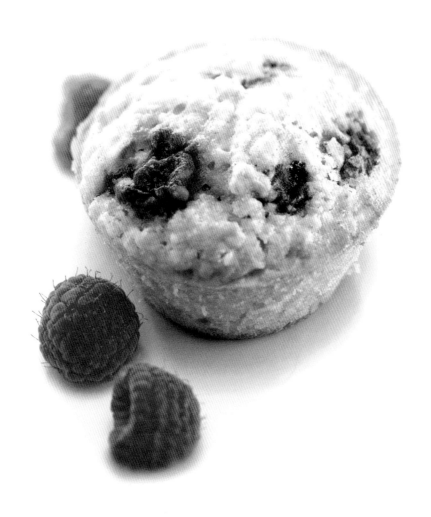

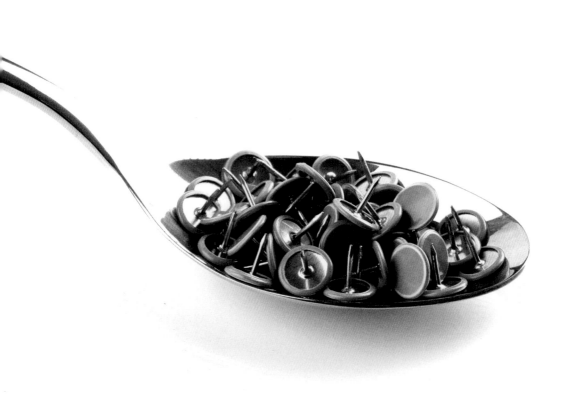

INTRODUCTION

Irritable bowel syndrome, or IBS, is an increasingly common health issue that manifests itself as abdominal pain, bowel dysfunction, bloating and excessive flatulence. These are all symptoms that occasionally disrupt the professional and domestic lives of the people affected, most of whom suffer in silence.

Irritable bowel syndrome is not a disease in itself. It is treated more as a functional disorder. Diet is therefore not considered a treatment. An adapted diet, however, helps to limit the symptoms (pain and discomfort), their duration and frequency, thus improving a person's quality of life.

Everyone reacts differently to foods. You need to learn to recognize the foods that agree with you and the foods that cause digestive problems. This book will help you identify these foods and create your own diet. Don't hesitate to consult a registered dietitian for help in adapting your diet to your physical condition while preventing nutritional deficiencies.

If you think you have a food allergy or an intolerance (for example, to gluten or lactose), or a more serious issue with symptoms that do not decrease, it is important not to self-diagnose but to see your doctor.

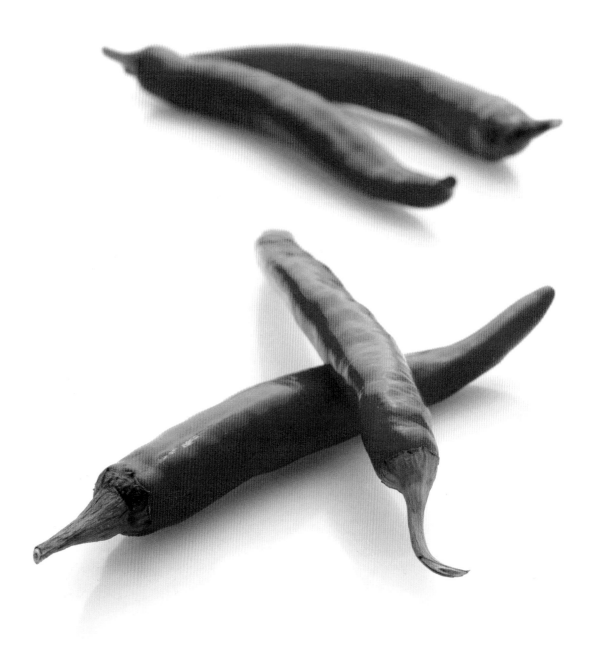

IRRITABLE BOWEL
Syndrome

Irritable bowel syndrome is associated with hypersensitivity in the intestinal wall and temperamental motility, or movement, in the colon, which can be at times overactive or underactive. Irritable bowel syndrome is not especially harmful to your health, but it produces pain and discomfort. Its underlying causes are little understood. It usually appears at the onset of adulthood, and women are generally more affected by it than men.

Irritable bowel syndrome is a functional disorder of the large intestine and not a type of allergy or food intolerance. Even if the symptoms are similar, IBS should not be confused with gluten or lactose intolerance, which are exclusively intolerances to one or the other substance. Irritable bowel syndrome encompasses multiple symptoms, including intolerance to various foods, and not just to gluten or lactose.

BIOLOGY 101

The principal functions of the large intestine (colon) are to store food residue and ensure that the body partially reabsorbs the water and nutrients in this residue. If intestinal transit time is too fast, less water is reabsorbed and stools become abnormally liquid, causing diarrhea. On the other hand, if intestinal transit time is too slow, the body reabsorbs too much water and stools become hard and dry, causing constipation.

When bacteria in the colon attacks the substances that the stomach and small intestine have not digested, intestinal gases are produced. This is a normal reaction. Some foods, however, contribute more than others to producing these intestinal gases. If a large quantity is produced, it causes bloating and an excessive amount of flatulence.

Fatigue, stress, a person's emotional state and even hormonal changes stimulate the nervous system, which in turn affect the digestive system. Again, this is a normal reaction, but IBS sufferers are more sensitive to these normal movements in the large intestine, which cause them pain.

SYMPTOMS OF IRRITABLE BOWEL SYNDROME

Irritable bowel syndrome is a chronic problem that can manifest itself in many ways.

FREQUENT SYMPTOMS	
• Pain, constipation	• Intestinal rumbling
• Diarrhea	• Mucus in the stools
• Bloating	• Flatulence
• Cramps	

LESS FREQUENT SYMPTOMS	
• Headaches	• Lower back pain
• Nausea, heartburn	• Sleeping problems
• Pelvic pain	

All these symptoms are recurrent and appear intermittently, with relatively long periods of remission in between. They are more likely to occur during periods of stress, and then generally following a meal. Symptoms are often absent upon awakening, becoming more pronounced as the day goes on.

Unlike many intestinal diseases, including ulcerative colitis and Crohn's disease, irritable bowel syndrome is a benign condition. It does not cause inflammation and does not damage the intestinal wall. It therefore does not increase the risk of colon cancer. Recurring symptoms such as diarrhea and constipation, however, can lead to specific problems in the long term, including dehydration and malnutrition.

GENERAL RECOMMENDATIONS

Except for symptomatic treatments, which, as their name suggests, are designed to ease symptoms, there are currently no medical solutions for treating irritable bowel syndrome. Remember that IBS is not a disease but a functional disorder.

Here are some tips for reducing symptoms:

AN ADAPTED DIET

The best treatment so far for irritable bowel syndrome is an adapted diet. It is important to understand that this syndrome does not manifest itself in the same way for everyone and that there are foods that agree with some individuals but not others. It is up to you to learn to recognize the foods you can tolerate and those you cannot. What's more, some foods may agree with you when you are feeling good, but may be less well tolerated during a crisis or period of stress. This is why a food should not necessarily be radically eliminated from your diet. Avoid both excesses and extreme restrictions. (See *Daily Nutritional Recommendations*, p. 15.)

PROPER STRESS MANAGEMENT

Many studies show that irritable bowel syndrome is linked to the sensitivity of people to normal movements in the large intestine, which are usually imperceptible. Stress activates these movements, even in individuals who do not appear to have gastrointestinal problems. Although stress is not recognized as a direct cause of the syndrome, it seems to accentuate the symptoms. Studies show that proper stress management helps to reduce the frequency, duration and gravity of symptoms in many people suffering from this syndrome.

Physical activity, relaxation and yoga are different ways to reduce and more effectively control one's stress. It is up to each individual to find daily remedies for getting rid of stress and managing frustration, for example, by having a bath, cooking or listening to music. Help from outside resources, such as psychotherapy, may also be useful.

A HEALTHIER LIFESTYLE

To help manage anxiety and prevent constipation, it is recommended that you do a half hour of physical exercise each day. Regular sleep cycles are also recommended. Finally, quitting smoking is strongly recommended, because nicotine is an aggravating factor.

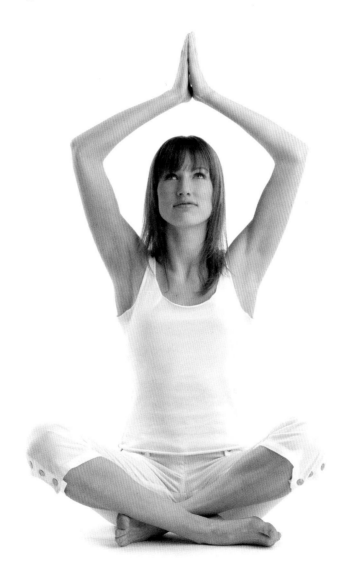

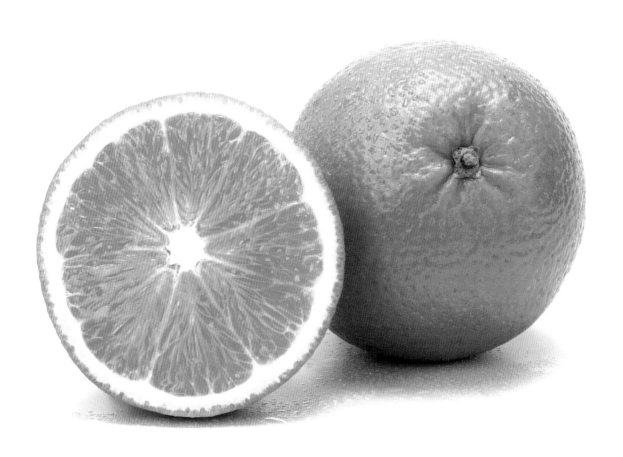

DAILY NUTRITIONAL
Recommendations

The recommendations made in this chapter are mainly designed to reduce hyper-stimulation and hyperdistension (major swelling) of the large intestine, which cause discomfort (abdominal pain, flatulence, gas and bowel dysfunction).

If you have doubts or if your symptoms remain unchecked, you are strongly advised to see your doctor and consult a registered dietitian to receive personalized advice.

RECOMMENDATIONS:

1. Temporarily adopt a low-FODMAP diet
2. Aim for a balanced diet at each meal
3. Have your meals at regular times each day
4. Drink a lot of water
5. Adopt a low-fat diet
6. Avoid very spicy foods
7. Reduce your consumption of refined sugar as much as possible
8. Limit your consumption of caffeine and alcohol

1 TEMPORARILY ADOPT A LOW-FODMAP DIET

FODMAP is an acronym referring to Fermentable Oligosaccharides, Disaccharides, Monosaccharides And Polyols. These are carbohydrates (sugars) present in foods such as wheat along with many other grain products, some fruits and vegetables, dairy products containing lactose and some sweetening agents. Foods that contain FODMAPs are fermentable by bacteria in the colon, which can cause digestive discomfort.

F for Fermentable

Oligosaccharides, disaccharides, monosaccharides and polyols are carbohydrates that are fermentable by intestinal flora.

O for Oligosaccharides

These carbohydrates are found in some vegetables (including artichokes, asparagus, beets, broccoli, Brussels sprouts, cabbage, fennel, garlic, green onions, onions and shallots), some grains (including barley, rye and wheat), some fruits (such as watermelon), legumes (including chickpeas, kidney beans, lentils and soybeans) and cashew nuts and pistachio nuts.

D for Disaccharides

Of all the disaccharides, lactose (the sugar in milk) causes the most digestive problems. Disaccharides are found in dairy products that come from cow's, sheep's and goat's milk.

M for Monosaccharides

These mainly include fructose (the sugar naturally found in fruit). It is problematic when there is an excessive amount of fructose in relation to glucose. The fruits with a high-fructose content are apples, figs, mangos, peaches, pears and watermelon.

A for And

P for Polyols

These are found in sweeteners (for example: sorbitol, mannitol and xylitol), some candy and other products labeled "sugar-free," some fruits (including apples, apricots, blackberries, cherries, nectarines, peaches, pears, plums, prunes and watermelon) and some vegetables (avocados, cauliflower, mushrooms and snow peas).

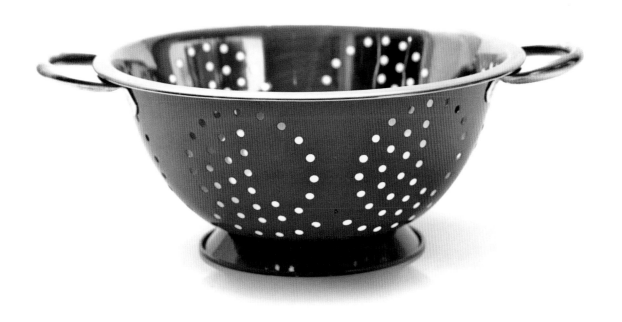

TEMPORARY REMOVAL OF HIGH-FODMAP FOODS

To help you manage your symptoms of irritable bowel syndrome, you should start by eliminating high-FODMAP foods from your diet for a period of six to eight weeks. The objective is to significantly reduce the quantity of FODMAPs you ingest, but not eliminate them completely.

It is not because FODMAPs are harmful to your health that it is recommended you reduce them as much as possible for several weeks — it is because some people with irritable bowel syndrome have difficulty digesting some of these sugars. The objective of this dietary restriction is to help identify which ones are at the origin of your digestive problems. Removing high-FODMAP foods gives your large intestine a chance to rest, thus reducing symptoms and discomfort. If you have difficulty following such a diet temporarily, you should meet with a registered dietitian to help you through the process.

It is important to understand that you do not have to follow a FODMAP-free diet, but a low-FODMAP diet — small quantities can be tolerated without causing particular symptoms. Most foods contain FODMAPs to some degree.

You should exclude those that have a high-FODMAP content (see *High-FODMAP Foods*, p. 19) and replace them with foods that have a low-FODMAP content (see *Low-FODMAP Foods*, p. 20). Foods that do not figure on either list should be limited during the elimination phase and reintroduced later.

All the recipes in this book are low in FODMAPs. They have been designed to help you cook easily and eat nutritiously without too many constraints during the elimination phase.

READ LABELS

Limit your consumption of commercially prepared products containing inulin or fructose, which are high in FODMAPs.

HIGH-FODMAP FOODS (TO AVOID)

Fruits	• Apples, apricots, blackberries, cherries, figs, mangos, nectarines, peaches, pears, plums, prunes, watermelon • Dried fruits, fruit juices
Vegetables	• Artichokes, asparagus, baby green peas, broccoli, Brussels sprouts, cauliflower, garlic, green onions (white part), leeks, mushrooms, onions, snow peas
Milk and Substitutes	• Cow's milk, goat's milk • Ice cream, yogurt • Soft cheeses (cottage cheese, cream cheese, goat cheese, mascarpone, ricotta,)
Grain Products	• Wheat-based breakfast cereals, cookies, croissants, muffins, pastries, wheat germ • Barley, bulgur, Kamut (khorasan wheat), rye • White flour, wheat flour, multigrain flour, all flours derived from grains listed above • All breads containing grains listed above • Pasta, including couscous • Breadcrumbs • Granola
Protein	• Legumes • Pistachio nuts, cashew nuts • Sausages and all other processed meats that contain onion, onion powder or garlic powder
Sugar and Sweeteners	• Honey, agave syrup, corn syrup • Sorbitol, mannitol, maltitol, xylitol
Other Products	• Relish, chutney, salad dressing, commercially prepared sauces • Onion powder and garlic powder

LOW-FODMAP FOODS (TO FAVOR)	
Fruits	• Bananas, blueberries, cantaloupes, cranberries, grapes, grapefruit, honeydew melons, kiwis, lemons, limes, mandarins, oranges, papaya, pineapple, passion fruits, raspberries, rhubarb, strawberries, tangerines
Vegetables	• Bean sprouts, bell peppers, bok choy, carrots, celery (in small quantities), Chinese cabbage, cucumbers, eggplant, green beans, lettuce, olives, parsnips, potatoes, pumpkin, rutabaga, green onions (green part), spinach, squash, tomatoes, turnip, zucchini
Milk and Substitutes	• Butter • Lactose-free milk, coconut milk, rice milk, soy milk • Ripened cheeses (feta, Parmesan, blue cheese, Brie, Gorgonzola, mozzarella), hard cheeses (Cheddar, Swiss, Emmental, Gouda, Gruyère) • Lactose-free yogurt, coconut milk yogurt • Lactose-free ice cream, low-fat sour cream
Grain Products	• Gluten-free cereals, rolled oats, tapioca, gluten-free breadcrumbs, popcorn • Gluten-free flour, gluten-free bread • Buckwheat, millet, quinoa, rice • Gluten-free pasta, gluten-free soba noodles, rice noodles

LOW-FODMAP FOODS (TO FAVOR)

Protein	• Beef (preferably lean), chicken, pork, eggs • Fish and seafood (at least twice a week) • Tofu • Nuts and seeds (except pistachio nuts and cashew nuts), nut butter
Sugar and sweeteners	• Aspartame, brown sugar, granulated sugar, maple syrup, molasses, stevia
Other products	• Oil, vinegar, mayonnaise, mustard, soy sauce, chili sauce that does not contain garlic • Ginger, spices and herbs (except onion powder and garlic powder) • Baking powder, cocoa, coconut, gelatin • Herbal tea, unflavored mineral water

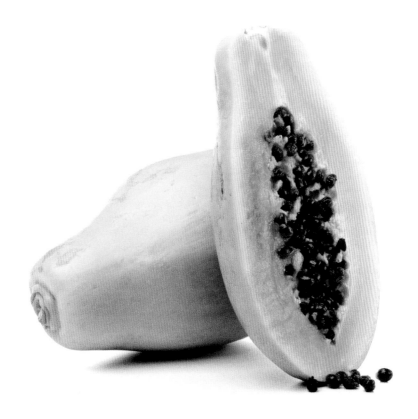

GLUTEN-FREE AND WHEAT-FREE

Gluten is a protein present in many grains, including wheat and barley. Celiac disease sufferers must absolutely eliminate all traces of gluten from their diet. For some irritable bowel syndrome sufferers, it is not gluten that causes their symptoms, but wheat, among other foods that are high in FODMAPs.

During the six-to-eight week phase of eliminating high-FODMAP foods, it is essential to remove wheat from the diet. It is easy to replace the food products that contain wheat with gluten-free products, which are available in an ever-growing range in grocery stores. For example, you can buy gluten-free bread, gluten-free pasta and gluten-free breakfast cereals. All of these products are wheat-free. Choosing products certified gluten-free is practical, because there are many more products labeled "gluten-free" than "wheat-free."

GLUTEN-FREE FLOUR

Many specialized boutiques and some grocery stores offer a choice of ready-to-use gluten-free flour mixes. It is a good idea to have gluten-free flour mixes at home to help you cook or bake more easily whenever you wish.

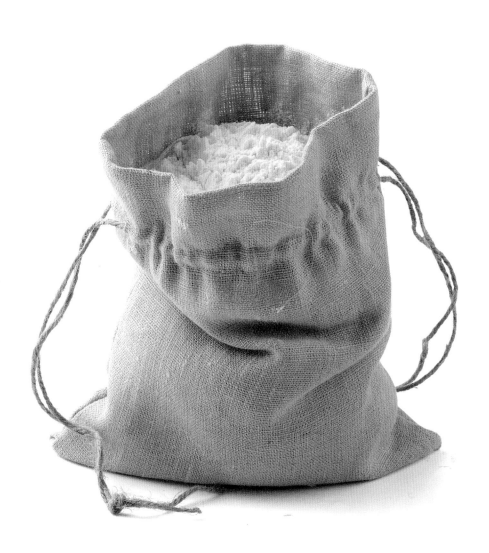

REINTRODUCING FOODS CONTAINING FODMAPS

After the six to eight week phase of eliminating high-FODMAP foods, you should see an improvement in your symptoms. You can then reintroduce certain foods gradually, but only one at a time, to see which ones you tolerate and which ones you should eliminate from your diet once and for all. Follow the recommendations listed below. Remember that to ensure a balanced diet, you must reintroduce as many foods as possible in the medium term, as long as you tolerate them. This will help you benefit from a diet that is as varied as possible.

It is important to be patient during the reintroduction phase and to proceed with one food at a time. If not, it will be very difficult to identify the foods that are causing problems and you could end up having to start all over again, removing all high-FODMAP foods from your diet for six to eight weeks.

If you don't have symptoms after introducing a food, you can consider it well tolerated and can go on to reintroduce another food.

If you have symptoms after introducing a food, you can reduce the serving and try it again to see if the symptoms persist. Alternatively, you can consider it problematic and eliminate it from your diet once and for all.

If your symptoms return, you can once again exclude foods containing FODMAPs from your diet for a few weeks, and then gradually reintroduce the foods that seem problematic. Don't forget that if you find this process arduous, you can ask for help from a professional registered dietitian.

RECOMMENDATIONS FOR GRADUALLY REINTRODUCING FOODS CONTAINING FODMAPS

- Reintroduce one food group at a time. For example, you can start with fruits. Once this entire group has been tested, go on to the next group. Do not reintroduce more than one food a day and no more than one food group a week.

- Eat a normal serving – one that you would normally consume (for example, one apple, one slice of bread or one glass of milk). Avoid exaggerating the quantities, because then you risk having symptoms and obtaining skewed results.

- Be aware of the cumulative effect of FODMAPs. The threshold of tolerance varies from one person to another.

- During the reintroduction phase, avoid consuming all other foods that are rich in FODMAPs that you have not already reintroduced.

Suggested order for reintroducing the different food groups:

1. Fruits

2. Dairy products

3. Vegetables

4. Grains

5. Legumes and nuts

6. Sugar and others

- Keep a food journal. As you progress, note the foods you have reintroduced, along with the symptoms, if any, or the absence of reaction to each food. It is very important to keep your journal up to date so that you don't forget which foods are problematic and which are not.

2 AIM FOR A BALANCED DIET AT EACH MEAL

Prepare a balanced dish for yourself at lunchtime and dinnertime. Choose a low-fat source of protein that will fill one quarter of your plate. This is sufficient to get the protein and nutrients you need.

Fill the other quarter of your plate with starches and grains.

Fill the remaining half of your plate with vegetables.

Have a snack if you are hungry in the morning, afternoon or evening.

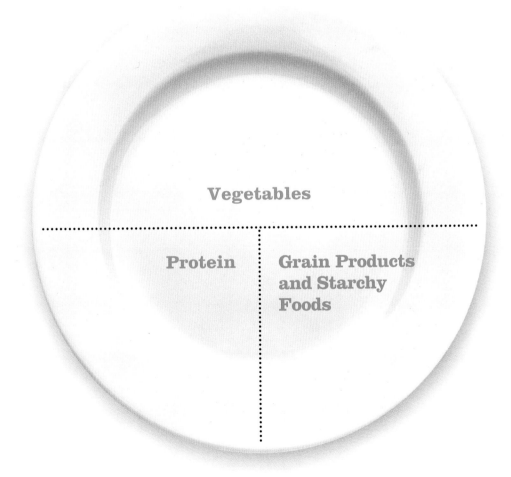

Vegetables

Protein

Grain Products
and Starchy
Foods

3 HAVE YOUR MEALS AT REGULAR TIMES EACH DAY

It is recommended that you eat three small meals a day, at regular times, and add three snacks if necessary, spread over the day.

Don't skip meals. On the other hand, avoid large meals that will overburden your digestive system. Plan to have a snack if you are worried about having hunger pangs.

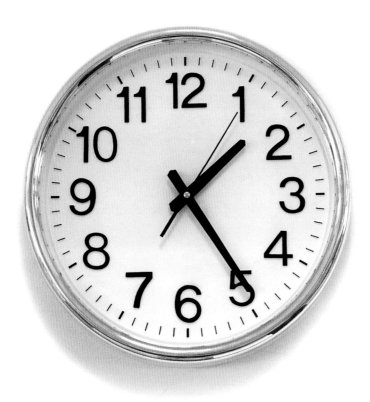

4 DRINK A LOT OF WATER

Water helps reduce the risk of constipation and keeps you properly hydrated, which is essential.

Drink a lot of water — at least 4 to 6 glasses (4 to 6 cups/1 to 1.5 liters) per day, preferably outside of mealtimes. Get into the habit of always having a bottle of water with you and drinking regularly throughout the day.

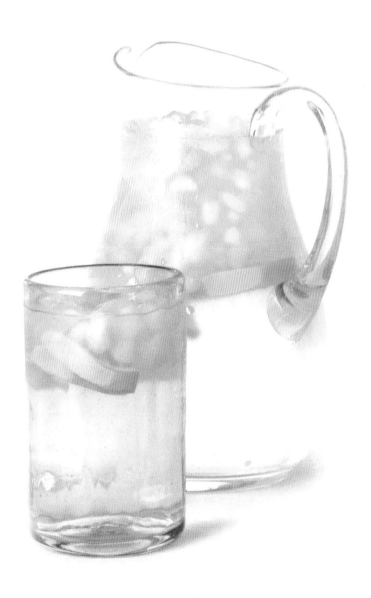

5 ADOPT A LOW-FAT DIET

It is recommended that you limit all sources of fat, whether they are unsaturated, saturated or trans fats. They slow down digestion and greatly stimulate contractions, or gastrocolic reflex, in the large intestine.

TIPS FOR LIMITING YOUR FAT CONSUMPTION

- Avoid fried foods, fatty meats and high-fat cheeses, dishes that contain a lot of oil, pâtés, chips and pastries.

- Choose lean meats (chicken, pork, lean beef, game, horse), fish, cheese containing less than 20% milk fat and milk containing 1% milk fat or less.

- Use nonstick saucepans and skillets as much as possible when cooking to limit your fat consumption.

- Add vegetable broth instead of oil or cream to sauces.

- Replace some oils with puréed fruit in your recipes for breads and cakes.

- Instead of baking chocolate use cocoa powder, which contains less fat.

6 AVOID VERY SPICY FOODS

Spicy foods can irritate the large intestine and cause discomfort. To liven up your dishes, replace spices (such as chili, Cajun, curry and other seasonings) with herbs (such as basil, mint, oregano, thyme, dill, cilantro, parsley).

Peppermint leaves may ease abdominal cramps, as they help intestinal muscles to relax. You can try consuming them in tea form.

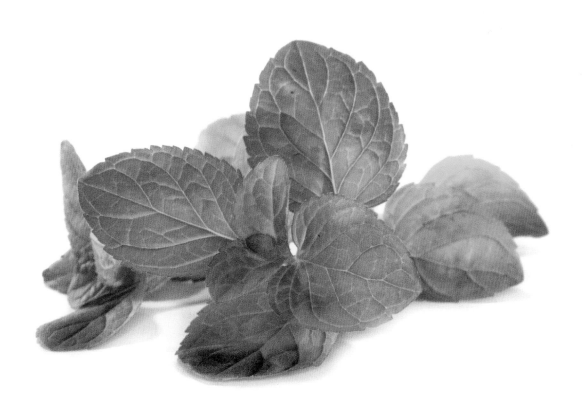

7 REDUCE YOUR CONSUMPTION OF REFINED SUGAR AS MUCH AS POSSIBLE

Excessive consumption of refined sugar can increase diarrhea and digestive discomfort.

Some foods rich in refined sugar to avoid

- Cookies, cakes, pies, ice cream and ice pops
- Carbonated beverages, sweetened juices and fruit cocktails
- Candy and chocolate bars
- Pastries

TIPS FOR REDUCING REFINED SUGAR IN YOUR DIET

- Don't add granulated sugar to your cereals and beverages. If you do, reduce the amount you normally add.

- Choose tap water over juices and carbonated beverages, even if they are labeled "diet."

- Prepare your own meals and snacks as often as possible, and reduce by half the amount of sugar called for in recipes. You can also use no-added-sugar applesauce to replace sugar in some recipes.

- Avoid commercially prepared desserts.

- Read nutrition labels to select products that contain less sugar.

8 LIMIT YOUR CONSUMPTION OF CAFFEINE AND ALCOHOL

Caffeine and theine stimulate activity in the large intestine and can cause diarrhea or discomfort. Avoid coffee, tea, caffeine-based energy drinks, chocolate and alcohol. They are acidic and can irritate the mucous membrane of the large intestine.

If you wish to drink these beverages from time to time, it is recommended that you have them with food. Don't drink coffee on an empty stomach in the morning and don't drink alcohol between meals or as an aperitif.

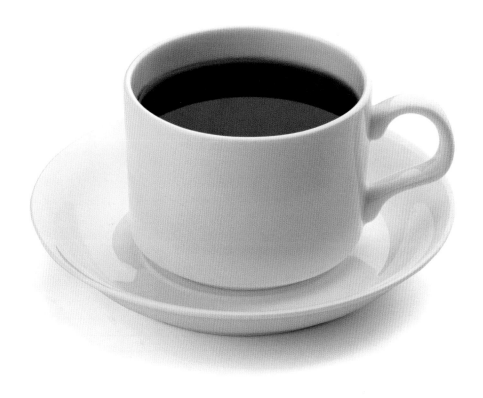

21 DAYS
OF MENUS

The menus in this book have been created to help you follow a low-FODMAP diet easily while meeting your body's nutritional requirements. You will find all of the recipes in the next chapter (see p. 59).

The meals and snacks are interchangeable from one day to ánother. You will also see that the lunchtime meals are often leftovers from the previous evening. You should therefore adjust recipe servings accordingly, doubling the amounts if necessary so that you have leftovers for the next day.

Snacks are an option and should only be eaten if you are hungry between meals. Trust your appetite to gauge the serving size to put on your plate. Try everything, but do not force yourself to finish everything on your plate if you are no longer hungry. If you have a small appetite, be sure to eat a variety of foods throughout the day, choosing from each of the three groups (protein, starches and grains, and vegetables) at every meal.

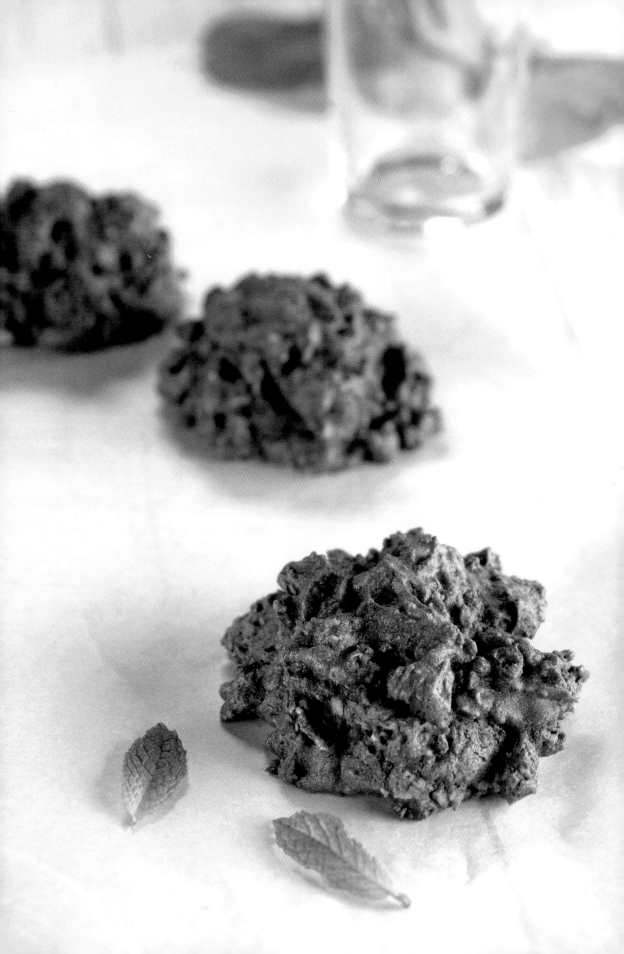

DAY 1

BREAKFAST

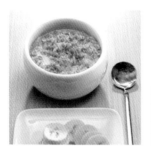

Omega-3 Oatmeal (p. 60)

Snack
2 clementines

LUNCH

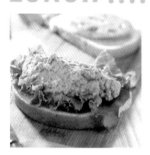

1 Salmon Mousse Sandwich (p. 84)
served with raw baby vegetables

Snack
1 lactose-free yogurt

DINNER

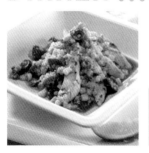

Mexican Quinoa Salad (p. 87)

Snack
1 orange

DAY 2

BREAKFAST

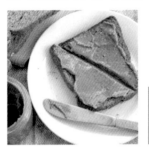

1 or 2 slices gluten-free bread
1 tbsp nut butter
½ cup (125 ml) blueberries

Snack
1 banana

LUNCH

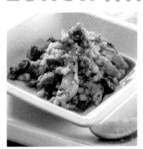

Mexican Quinoa Salad (p. 87)

Snack
1 Raspberry Muffin (p. 74)

DINNER

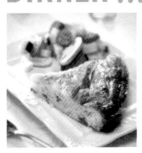

Bell Pepper Quiche (p. 88)
served with a baby vegetable salad

Snack
½ cup (125 ml) gluten-free oat cereal
½ cup (125 ml) lactose-free milk
or plain soy milk

DAY 3

BREAKFAST . . . .

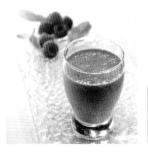

1 Choco-Banana Smoothie (p. 62)
1 Raspberry Muffin (p. 74)

Snack
½ cup (125 ml) berries

LUNCH . . . .

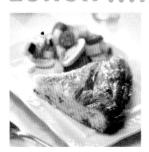

Bell Pepper Quiche (p. 88)
served with a baby vegetable salad

Snack
1 lactose-free yogurt

DINNER . . . .

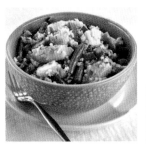

Herbed Sole Casserole (p. 90)

Snack
½ cup (125 ml) pineapple

DAY 4

BREAKFAST

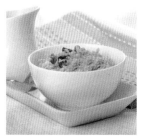

¾ cup (180 ml) gluten-free oat cereal
½ cup (125 ml) lactose-free milk or plain soy milk
1 banana

Snack
1 Choco-Mint Cookie (p. 77)

LUNCH

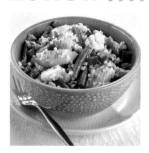

Herbed Sole Casserole (p. 90)

Snack
1 orange

DINNER

Beef and Rice Soup (p. 92)

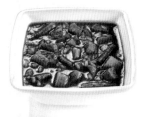

Snack
1 lactose-free yogurt
2 small gluten-free social tea biscuits

DAY 5

BREAKFAST

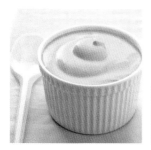

¾ cup (180 ml) lactose-free yogurt
½ cup (125 ml) fresh fruit
1 slice gluten-free bread

Snack
1 lactose-free yogurt

LUNCH

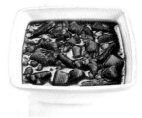

Beef and Rice Soup (p. 92)

Snack
½ cup (125 ml) pineapple

DINNER

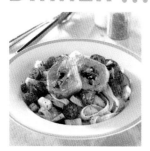

Pork Stuffed with Olives (p. 94)
served with fettuccini and zucchini

Snack
1 Raspberry Muffin (p. 74)
½ cup (125 ml) lactose-free milk
or plain soy milk

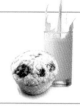

DAY 6

BREAKFAST ....

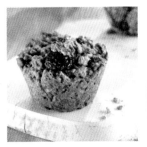

1 Spiced Strawberry Muffin (p. 78)
1 cup (250 ml) lactose-free milk or plain soy milk
½ cup (125 ml) kiwi

Snack
1 lactose-free yogurt

LUNCH ....

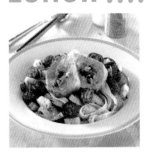

Pork Stuffed with Olives (p. 94)
served with fettuccini and zucchini

Snack
1 Choco-Mint Cookie (p. 77)

DINNER ....

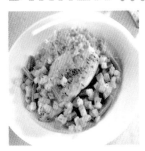

Pineapple Chicken (p. 96)
served with brown rice

Snack
1 banana

DAY 7

BREAKFAST . . . .

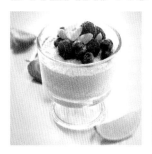

1 Energy Breakfast (p. 64)

Snack
1 orange

LUNCH . . . .

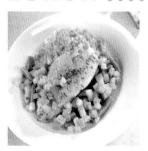

Pineapple Chicken (p. 96)
served with brown rice

Snack
1 oz (30 g) low-fat Cheddar cheese
½ cup (125 ml) raspberries

DINNER . . . .

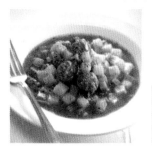

Easy Stew (p. 98)

Snack
2 cups (500 ml) homemade popcorn

43

DAY 8

BREAKFAST ....

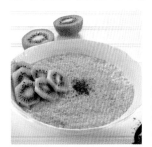

Cream of Oats (p. 66)
½ cup (125 ml) kiwi

Snack
½ cup (125 ml) berries

LUNCH ....

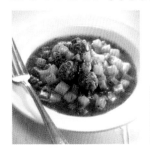

Easy Stew (p. 98)

Snack
1 lactose-free yogurt

DINNER ....

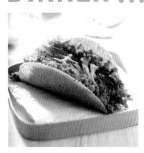

Egg Tacos (p. 100)

Snack
½ cup (125 ml) lactose-free milk
or plain soy milk

1 banana

DAY 9

BREAKFAST

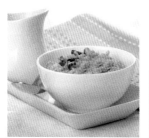

¾ cup (180 ml) gluten-free oat cereal
½ cup (125 ml) lactose-free milk or plain soy milk
1 banana

Snack
1 Banana and Almond Butter Cookie
(p. 80)

LUNCH

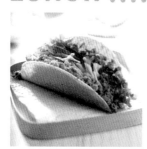

Egg Tacos (p. 100)

Snack
½ cup (125 ml) pineapple

DINNER

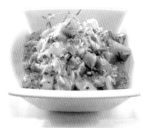

Simmered Chicken (p. 102)

Snack
1 lactose-free yogurt
2 small gluten-free social tea biscuits

DAY 10

BREAKFAST . . . .

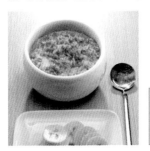

Omega-3 Oatmeal (p. 60)

Snack
½ cup (125 ml) berries

LUNCH . . . .

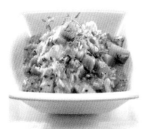

Simmered Chicken (p. 102)

Snack
1 lactose-free yogurt

DINNER . . . .

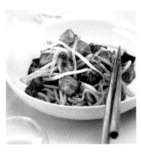

Salmon with Soba Noodles (p. 105)

Snack
1 Banana and Almond Butter Cookie
(p. 80)

DAY 11

BREAKFAST

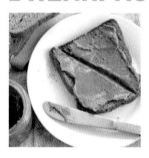

1 or 2 slices gluten-free bread
1 tbsp nut butter
½ cup (125 ml) blueberries

Snack
1 banana

LUNCH

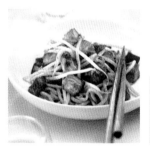

Salmon with Soba Noodles (p. 105)

Snack
1 Banana and Almond Butter Cookie
(p. 80)

DINNER

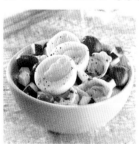

Meal Salad (p. 106)

Snack
1 lactose-free yogurt

DAY 12

BREAKFAST

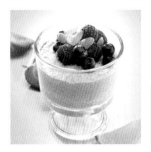

1 Energy Breakfast (p. 64)

Snack
1 orange

LUNCH

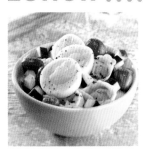

Meal Salad (p. 106)

Snack
1 lactose-free yogurt

DINNER

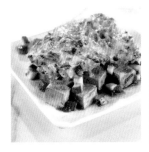

Vegetarian Casserole (p. 108)
served with quinoa or rice

Snack
½ cup (125 ml) gluten-free oat cereal
½ cup (125 ml) lactose-free milk
or plain soy milk

DAY 13

BREAKFAST . . . .

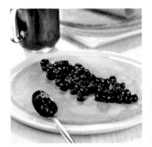

1 or 2 Blueberry Crêpes (p. 68)

Snack
1 Raspberry Muffin (p. 74)

LUNCH . . . .

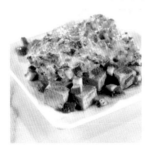

Vegetarian Casserole (p. 108)
served with quinoa or rice

Snack
2 clementines

DINNER . . . .

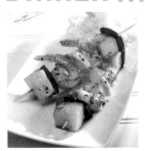

Shrimp Brochettes (p. 110)
served with jasmine rice

Snack
2 cups (500 ml) homemade popcorn

DAY 14

BREAKFAST

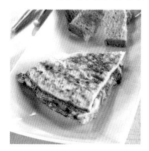

Morning Omelet (p. 70)
1 or 2 slices gluten-free bread
1 orange

Snack
½ cup (125 ml) pineapple

LUNCH

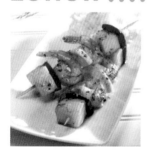

Shrimp Brochettes (p. 110)
served with jasmine rice

Snack
1 Choco-Mint Cookie (p. 77)

DINNER

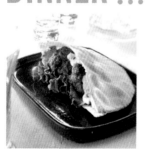

Veal Pita Pockets with Tzatziki (p. 113)

Snack
1 lactose-free yogurt
2 small gluten-free social tea biscuits

DAY 15

BREAKFAST ....

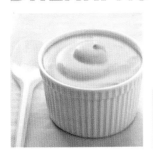

¾ cup (180 ml) lactose-free yogurt
½ cup (125 ml) fresh fruit
1 slice gluten-free bread

Snack
1 banana

LUNCH ....

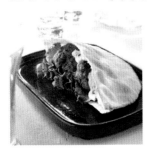

Veal Pita Pockets with Tzatziki (p. 113)

Snack
1 Choco-Mint Cookie (p. 77)
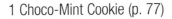

DINNER ....

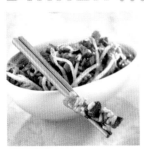

Chinese-Style Pork and Rice (p. 114)
served with bell peppers and bean sprouts

Snack
½ cup (125 ml) lactose-free yogurt
with a drizzle of maple syrup

DAY 16

BREAKFAST

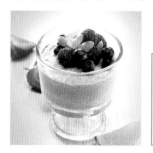

Energy Breakfast (p. 64)

Snack
¼ cup (60 ml) Granola with
Dried Bananas (p. 82)

1 lactose-free yogurt

LUNCH

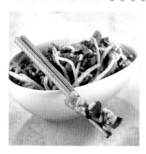

Chinese-Style Pork and Rice (p. 114)
served with bell peppers and bean sprouts

Snack
1 orange

DINNER

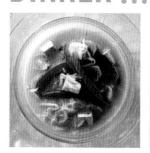

Asian Soup (p. 116)

Snack
½ cup (125 ml) lactose-free milk
or plain soy milk

2 small gluten-free social tea biscuits

DAY 17

BREAKFAST ....

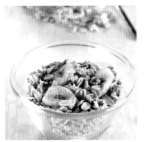

¼ cup (60 ml) Granola with Dried Banana Chips (p. 82)
¾ cup (180 ml) lactose-free yogurt
½ cup (125 ml) berries

Snack
1 Raspberry Muffin (p. 74)

LUNCH ....

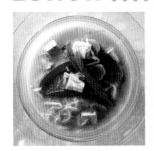

Asian Soup (p. 116)

Snack
2 kiwis

DINNER ....

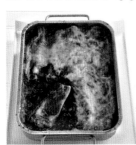

Cheese Cannelloni (p. 118)

Snack
1 Banana and
Almond Butter Cookie (p. 80)

DAY 18

BREAKFAST

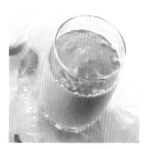

1 Pink Smoothie (p. 72)
1 Spiced Strawberry Muffin (p. 78)

Snack
1 banana

LUNCH

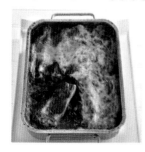

Cheese Cannelloni (p. 118)

Snack
1 Banana and Almond Butter Cookie
(p. 80)

DINNER

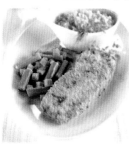

Breaded Fish (p. 120)
served with millet, carrots and green beans

Snack
¼ cup (60 ml) Granola
with Dried Banana Chips (p. 82)

¾ cup (180 ml) lactose-free yogurt

DAY 19

BREAKFAST

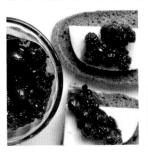

1 or 2 slices gluten-free bread
1 oz (30 g) low-fat Cheddar cheese
1 tbsp reduced-sugar jam

> **Snack**
> ½ cup (125 ml) pineapple

LUNCH

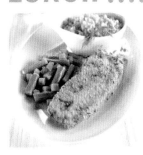

Breaded Fish (p. 120)
served with millet, carrots and green beans

> **Snack**
> ½ cup (125 ml) lactose-free yogurt
> with a drizzle of maple syrup

DINNER

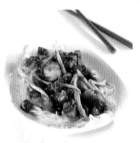

Chicken in Peanut Sauce (p. 122)
served with rice vermicelli and bell peppers

> **Snack**
> ½ cup (125 ml) lactose-free milk
> or plain soy milk
>
> 1 banana

DAY 20

BREAKFAST

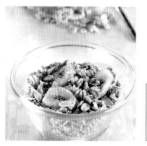

¼ cup (60 ml) Granola with Dried Banana Chips (p. 82)
¾ cup (180 ml) lactose-free yogurt

Snack
2 clementines

LUNCH

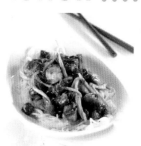

Chicken in Peanut Sauce (p. 122)
served with rice vermicelli and bell peppers

Snack
1 Choco-Mint Cookie (p. 77)

DINNER

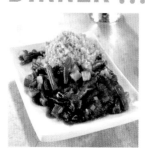

Beef with Vegetables (p. 125)
served with quinoa, zucchini and green beans

Snack
½ cup (125 ml) gluten-free oat cereal

½ cup (125 ml) lactose-free milk
or plain soy milk

DAY 21

BREAKFAST ....

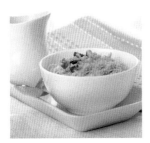

¾ cup (180 ml) gluten-free oat cereal
½ cup (125 ml) lactose-free milk or plain soy milk
1 banana

Snack
½ cup (125 ml) berries

LUNCH ....

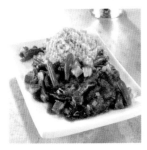

Beef with Vegetables (p. 125)
served with quinoa, zucchini and green beans

Snack
1 Banana and Almond Butter Cookie
(p. 80)
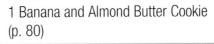

DINNER ....

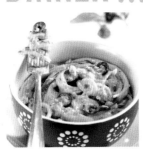

Linguini with Olives (p. 126)
served with baby spinach leaves

Snack
½ cup (125 ml) lactose-free yogurt
with a drizzle of maple syrup

RECIPES
34 HEALTHY IDEAS

Throughout this chapter, you will find DIGESTIVE HEALTH INFO boxes on many foods and how they benefit intestinal health and digestion.

OMEGA-3
Oatmeal

1 serving • PREPARATION: 5 minutes • COOKING TIME: 3 minutes

INGREDIENTS

½ cup (125 ml) old-fashioned rolled oats

¾ cup (180 ml) lactose-free milk or plain soy milk

1 tbsp chia seeds

1 tsp maple syrup

½ banana, sliced

METHOD

In a microwave-safe bowl, combine rolled oats, milk, chia seeds and maple syrup.

Cook in microwave for 3 minutes, stirring after each minute.

Add banana slices.

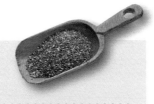

DIGESTIVE HEALTH INFO

• •

The chia seed promotes digestive health. Its high protein content makes it very nourishing. It is also a good source of omega-3 fatty acids, which help reduce inflammation.

Nutrition Facts
Per serving

Amount	
Calories	254
Fat	6 g
Sodium	90 mg
Carbohydrates	40 g
Fiber	6 g
Protein	11 g

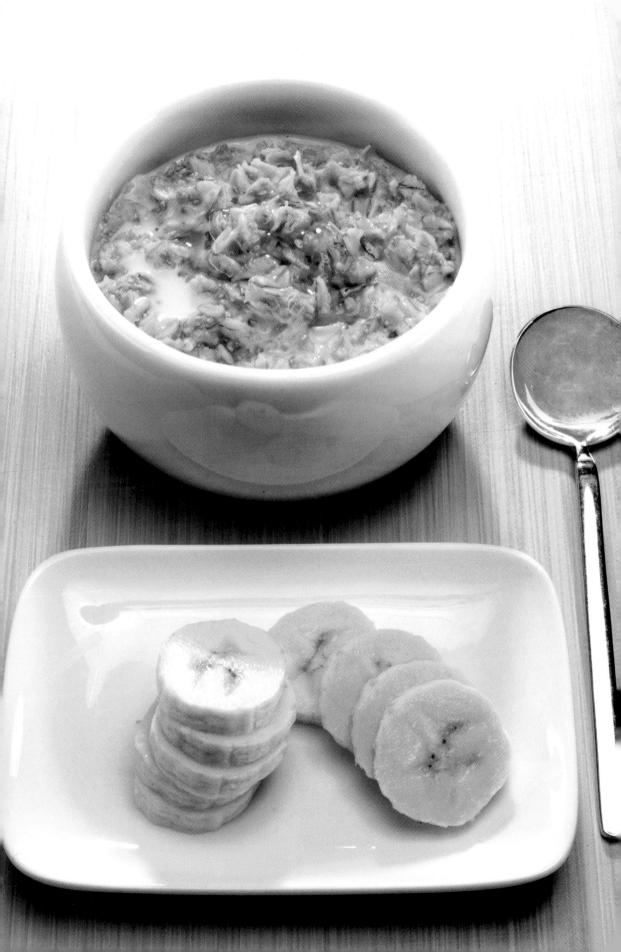

CHOCO-BANANA
Smoothie

2 smoothies • PREPARATION: 5 minutes

INGREDIENTS

½ cup (125 ml) lactose-free plain or coconut milk yogurt

½ cup (125 ml) lactose-free milk

½ banana, sliced

1 tbsp maple syrup

1 tbsp unsweetened cocoa powder

METHOD

In a blender or food processor, combine all ingredients and blend to a smooth, even consistency.

Serve chilled.

. . . .

TIP

Bananas freeze very well. Remove peels and place them in the freezer in an airtight bag or container.

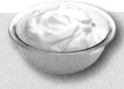

DIGESTIVE HEALTH INFO

Lactose-free yogurt contains calcium and is a good source of protein. It naturally contains probiotics, which are good bacteria recommended for digestive health. For a healthy choice, look for natural or plain yogurt with no added sugar or food additives.

Nutrition Facts
Per smoothie

Amount	
Calories	126
Fat	2 g
Sodium	75 mg
Carbohydrates	23 g
Fiber	2 g
Protein	7 g

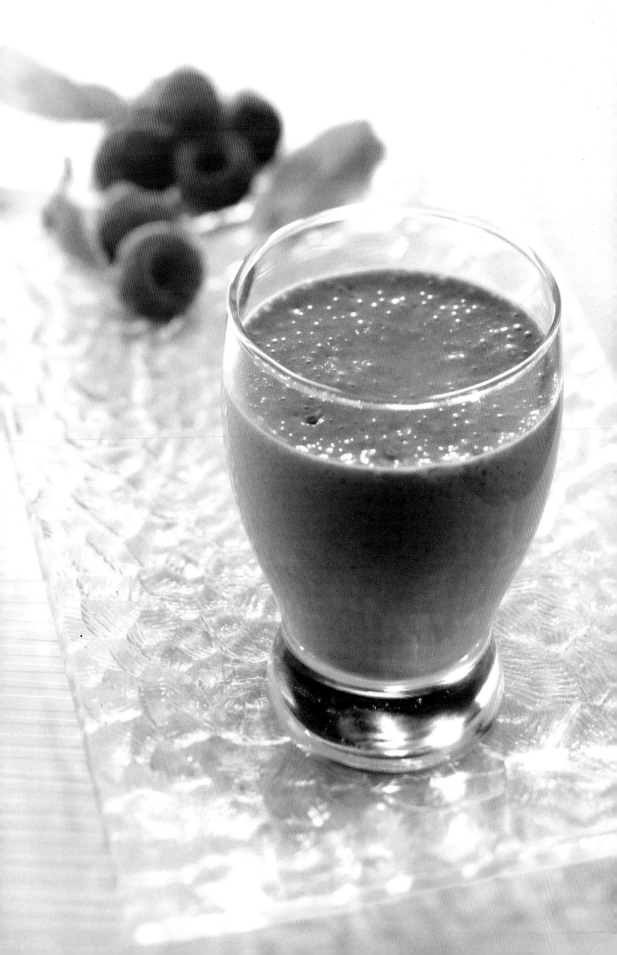

ENERGY
Breakfast

1 serving • PREPARATION: 5 minutes • RESTING TIME: 15 minutes

INGREDIENTS

¼ cup (60 ml) lactose-free plain or coconut milk yogurt

1 tsp maple syrup

¼ cup (60 ml) 100% pure orange juice

¼ cup (60 ml) chia seeds

1 tbsp slivered almonds

½ cup (125 ml) berries (blueberries, strawberries, raspberries)

Juice of ½ lime

METHOD

In a bowl, combine yogurt, maple syrup, orange juice and chia seeds. Let sit for 15 minutes.

Stir and garnish with almonds and berries. Drizzle with lime juice.

• • • • • • • • • • • • • •

TIP

Chia seeds keep well stored in an airtight container in your pantry.

Nutrition Facts
Per serving

Amount	
Calories	369
Fat	19 g
Sodium	55 mg
Carbohydrates	40 g
Fiber	20 g
Protein	13 g

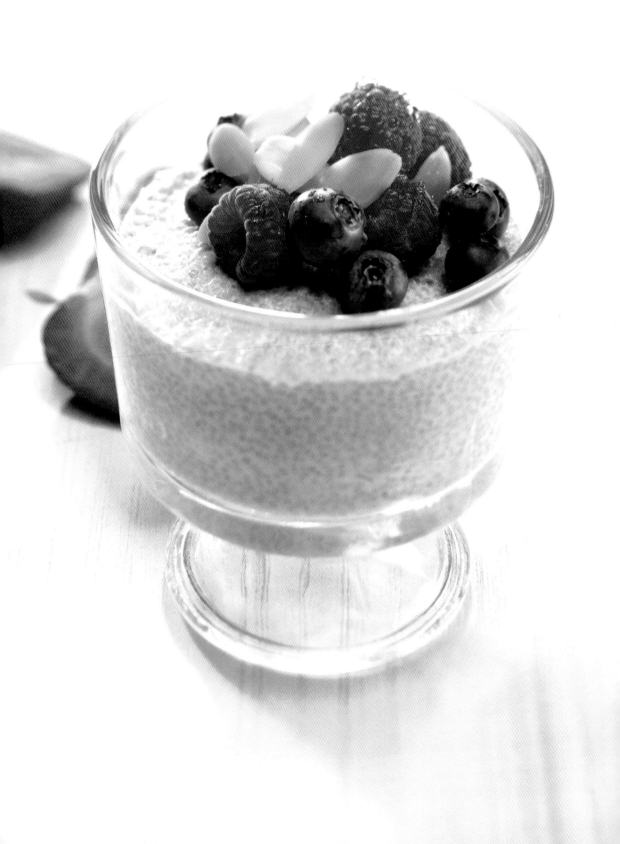

CREAM
of Oats

1 serving • PREPARATION: 5 minutes • COOKING TIME: 2 minutes

INGREDIENTS

½ cup (125 ml) oat bran

1 tsp brown sugar

½ cup (125 ml) lactose-free milk
or plain soy milk

¼ cup (60 ml) water

1 tbsp ground flaxseeds (optional)

2 kiwis, sliced

METHOD

In a microwave-safe bowl, combine oat bran, brown sugar, milk and water. Cook in microwave for 1 to 2 minutes.

Add flaxseeds, if using, and kiwi slices.

• • • • • • • • • • • • • •

VARIATION

Replace kiwis with other low-FODMAP fruits you have on hand (see p. 20).

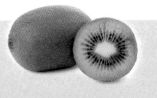

DIGESTIVE HEALTH INFO

• •

The kiwi is an excellent choice for breakfast or a snack. It is a good source of natural sugar, which helps to curb hunger and control sugar cravings.

Nutrition Facts
Per serving

Amount	
Calories	372
Fat	9 g
Sodium	67 mg
Carbohydrates	62 g
Fiber	14 g
Protein	13 g

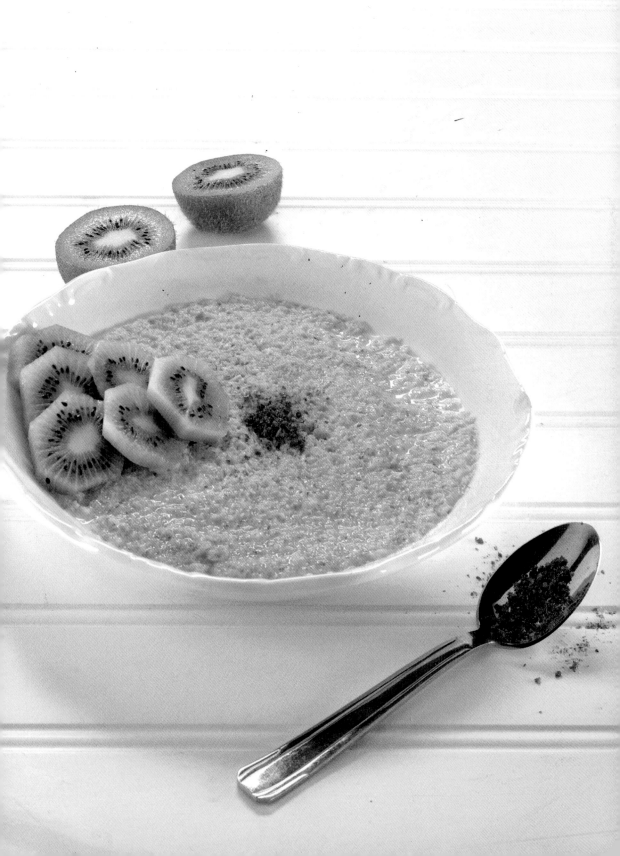

BLUEBERRY
Crêpes

6 crêpes • PREPARATION: 10 minutes • COOKING TIME: 20 minutes

INGREDIENTS

1½ cups (375 ml) gluten-free flour

¼ cup (60 ml) oat bran

3 eggs

2 cups (500 ml) lactose-free milk
or plain soy milk

1 tsp vanilla extract

Zest of ½ lemon

4 cups (1 liter) frozen blueberries

2 tbsp maple syrup

METHOD

In a bowl, combine flour, oat bran, eggs, milk, vanilla and lemon zest. Beat thoroughly to eliminate lumps.

In a preheated lightly oiled skillet over medium heat, pour one small ladle of batter and cook 6 thin crêpes, one at a time, for 3 to 4 minutes each.

Meanwhile, in another skillet over medium heat, heat blueberries and maple syrup, stirring frequently, for 10 minutes.

Spread filling on crêpes. Roll up crêpes and drizzle additional maple syrup on top, if desired.

• • • • • • • • • • • • •

TIP

Prepare your crêpes and, once they have cooled, place them in a resealable bag, separated individually by a sheet of waxed paper. Store in the freezer. Defrost in the microwave when you need them, heating for 30 seconds on each side.

Nutrition Facts Per crêpe	
Amount	
Calories	351
Fat	5 g
Sodium	74 mg
Carbohydrates	66 g
Fiber	8 g
Protein	11 g

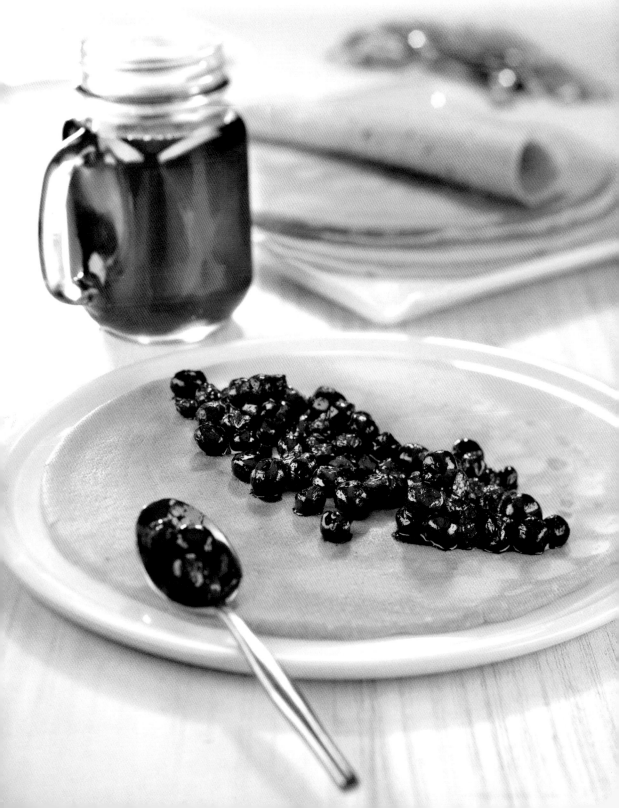

Omelet

4 servings • PREPARATION: 10 minutes • COOKING TIME: 10 minutes

INGREDIENTS

8 eggs

½ cup (125 ml) lactose-free milk

1 cup (250 ml) chopped spinach

1 cup (250 ml) grated Swiss cheese

For the seasonings

1 tbsp dried basil

Salt and black pepper

METHOD

In a bowl, using a fork, beat eggs with milk and seasonings.

Pour mixture into a preheated lightly oiled skillet. Cook over medium heat for 7 to 8 minutes or until omelet sets.

Top omelet with spinach and cheese, then fold in half. Continue to cook for 2 to 3 minutes without turning omelet over.

Serve with 1 or 2 slices of gluten-free bread.

Nutrition Facts Per serving	
Amount	
Calories	214
Fat	7 g
Sodium	223 mg
Carbohydrates	4 g
Fiber	0 g
Protein	22 g

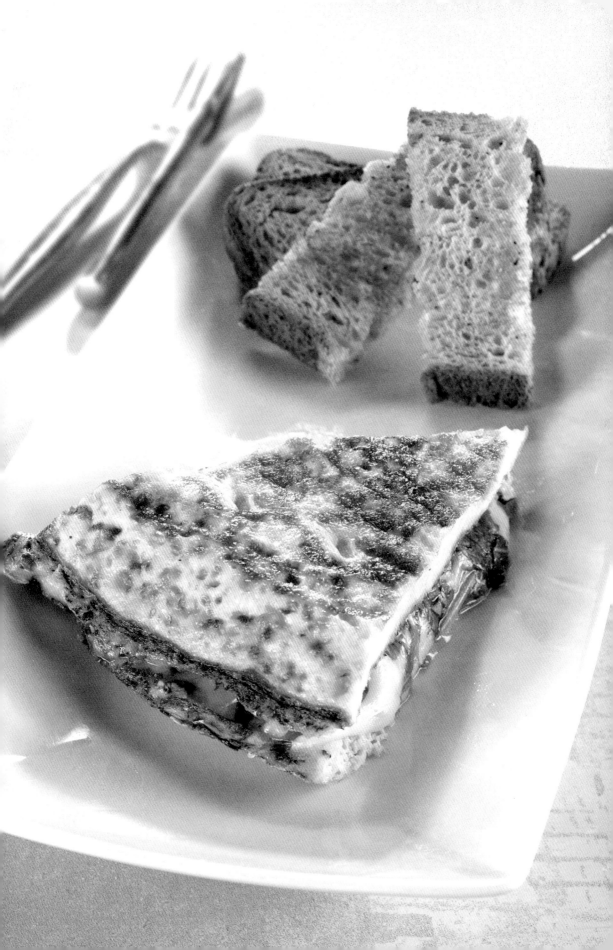

PINK
Smoothie

2 smoothies • PREPARATION: 5 minutes

INGREDIENTS

6 oz (180 g) soft silken tofu

1 cup (250 ml) fresh or frozen raspberries

1 cup (250 ml) lactose-free vanilla yogurt or coconut milk yogurt

1 tbsp maple syrup

METHOD

In a blender or food processor, combine all ingredients and blend to a smooth, even consistency.

Serve chilled.

• • • • • • • • • • • • •

VARIATION

Replace raspberries with blueberries, strawberries, pineapple or any other low-FODMAP fruit (see p. 20).

• • • • • • • • • • • • •

TIP

Freeze your fruits that are no longer very attractive. Lay them on a pastry sheet to freeze, then store in a resealable airtight bag. It's a good way to avoid waste and always have fruit on hand for making smoothies.

Nutrition Facts
Per smoothie

Amount	
Calories	190
Fat	4 g
Sodium	85 mg
Carbohydrates	28 g
Fiber	4 g
Protein	12 g

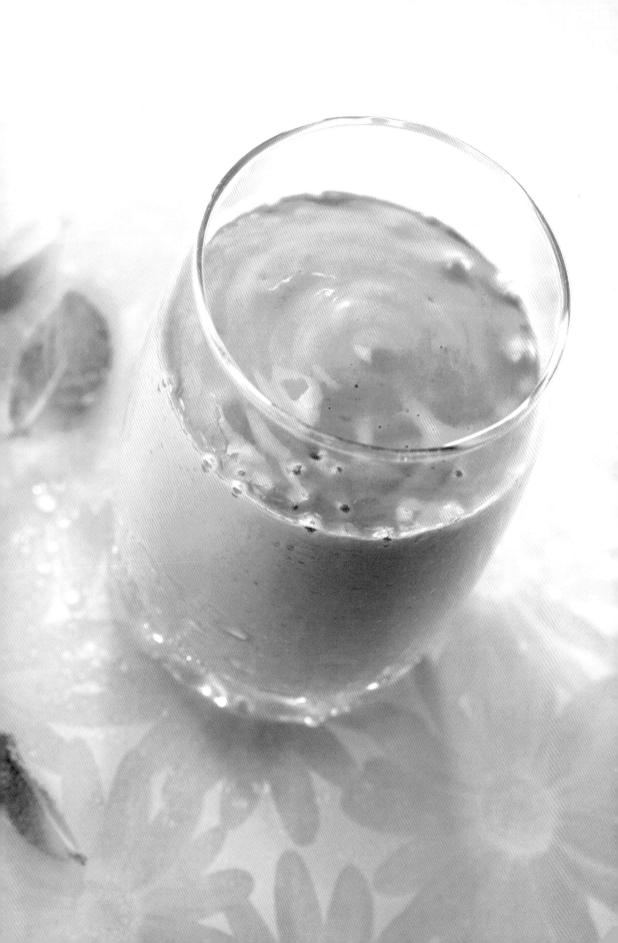

RASPBERRY
Muffins

12 muffins • PREPARATION: 10 minutes • COOKING TIME: 25 minutes

INGREDIENTS

1 cup (250 ml) gluten-free pastry flour mix

1 cup (250 ml) quick-cooking rolled oats

¼ cup (60 ml) oat bran

2 tsp baking powder

¼ cup (60 ml) canola oil

¼ cup (60 ml) sugar

2 eggs

1 cup (250 ml) lactose-free milk or plain soy milk

1½ cups (375 ml) frozen raspberries

METHOD

Place oven rack in center of oven and preheat to 350°F (180°C).

In a bowl, combine flour, rolled oats, oat bran and baking powder.

In another bowl, whisk together oil, sugar and eggs for 2 minutes. Add milk gradually while continuing to whisk ingredients.

Add dry ingredients to wet mixture, then add raspberries.

Pour mixture into an oiled or nonstick muffin pan and bake in preheated oven on middle rack for 20 to 25 minutes or until a toothpick inserted in the center comes out clean. Let cool on a rack.

. . . .

TIP

To save time, prepare a large quantity of muffins and freeze them in a resealable airtight bag. When you want a muffin, let it thaw at room temperature or reheat in the microwave for 15 to 20 seconds.

Nutrition Facts
Per muffin

Amount	
Calories	150
Fat	7 g
Sodium	70 mg
Carbohydrates	19 g
Fiber	2 g
Protein	4 g

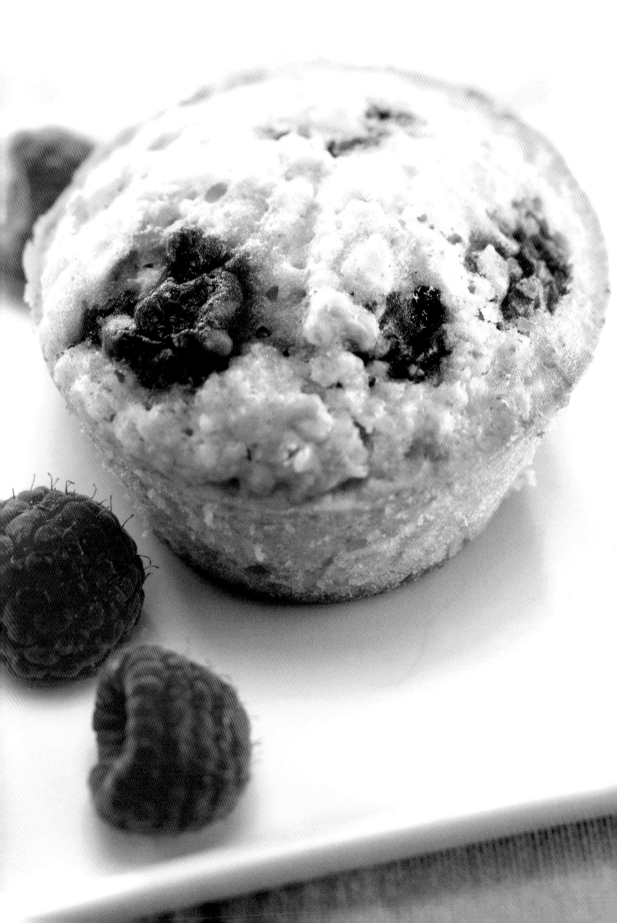

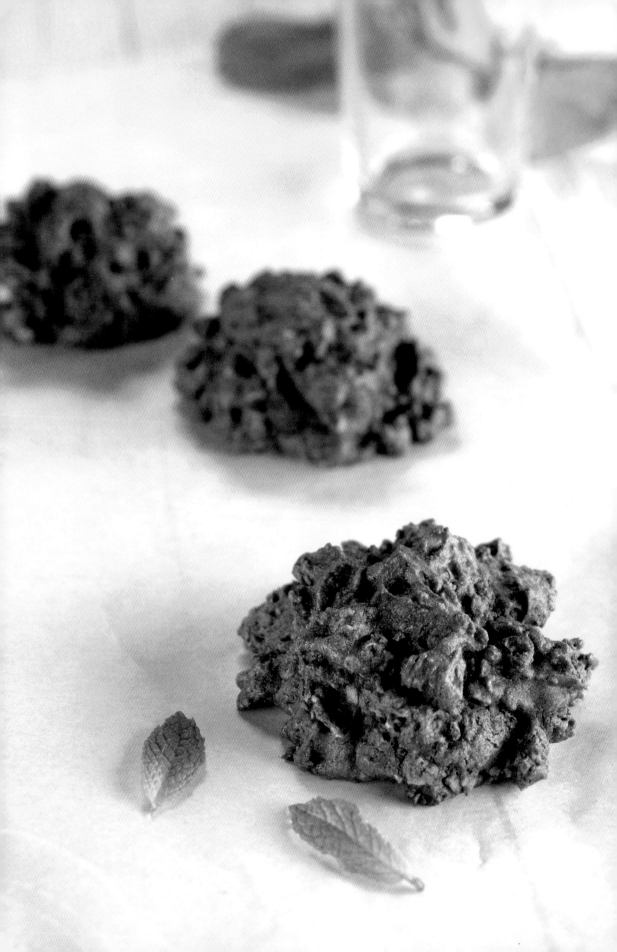

CHOCO-MINT
Cookies

12 cookies • PREPARATION: 10 minutes • COOKING TIME: 10 minutes

METHOD

Position rack in center of oven and preheat to 350°F (180°C). Line a baking sheet with parchment paper.

In a bowl, combine flour, rolled oats and cocoa powder.

In another bowl, beat together egg, brown sugar and butter. Add mint extract and milk. Add dry ingredients and mix together thoroughly.

On prepared baking sheet, drop 2 tbsp of dough per cookie to form 12 cookies.

Bake on middle rack in preheated oven for 8 minutes. Let cool on a rack.

INGREDIENTS

1 cup (250 ml) gluten-free pastry flour mix

1 cup (250 ml) quick-cooking rolled oats

¼ cup (60 ml) unsweetened cocoa powder

1 egg

½ cup (125 ml) brown sugar

¼ cup (60 ml) butter at room temperature

1 tsp mint extract

½ cup (125 ml) lactose-free milk or plain soy milk

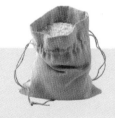

DIGESTIVE HEALTH INFO

• •

More and more specialized stores and supermarkets are offering ready-to-use gluten-free flour mixes. This is a good buy that will help people suffering with irritable bowel syndrome prepare desserts and nutritious snacks more easily.

Nutrition Facts	
Per cookie	
Amount	
Calories	154
Fat	6 g
Sodium	14 mg
Carbohydrates	22 g
Fiber	1 g
Protein	4 g

SPICED
Strawberry Muffins

12 muffins • PREPARATION: 20 minutes • COOKING TIME: 20 minutes

INGREDIENTS

1½ cups (375 ml) gluten-free pastry flour mix

1 cup (250 ml) quick-cooking rolled oats

2 tsp baking powder

1 tsp baking soda

¼ cup brown sugar

½ cup (125 ml) hemp seeds (or your choice of seeds)

2 tsp ground nutmeg

¼ tsp ground clove

1 egg

¾ cup (180 ml) lactose-free milk or plain soy milk

¼ cup (60 ml) canola oil

1 cup (250 ml) frozen strawberries, sliced

METHOD

Position rack in center of oven and preheat to 375°F (190°C).

In a bowl, combine flour, rolled oats, baking powder, baking soda, brown sugar, hemp seeds, nutmeg and clove.

In a large bowl, using a hand mixer, combine egg, milk and oil. Add strawberries and mix gently with a spoon.

Add dry ingredient mixture to wet mixture.

Pour mixture into an oiled or nonstick muffin pan and bake on middle rack in preheated oven for 15 to 20 minutes or until a toothpick inserted in the center comes out clean. Let cool on a rack.

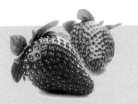

DIGESTIVE HEALTH INFO

The strawberry is a low-FODMAP fruit. It is a good source of vitamin C to add to recipes or simply to have as a snack.

Nutrition Facts Per muffin	
Amount	
Calories	183
Fat	9 g
Sodium	68 mg
Carbohydrates	21 g
Fiber	4 g
Protein	5 g

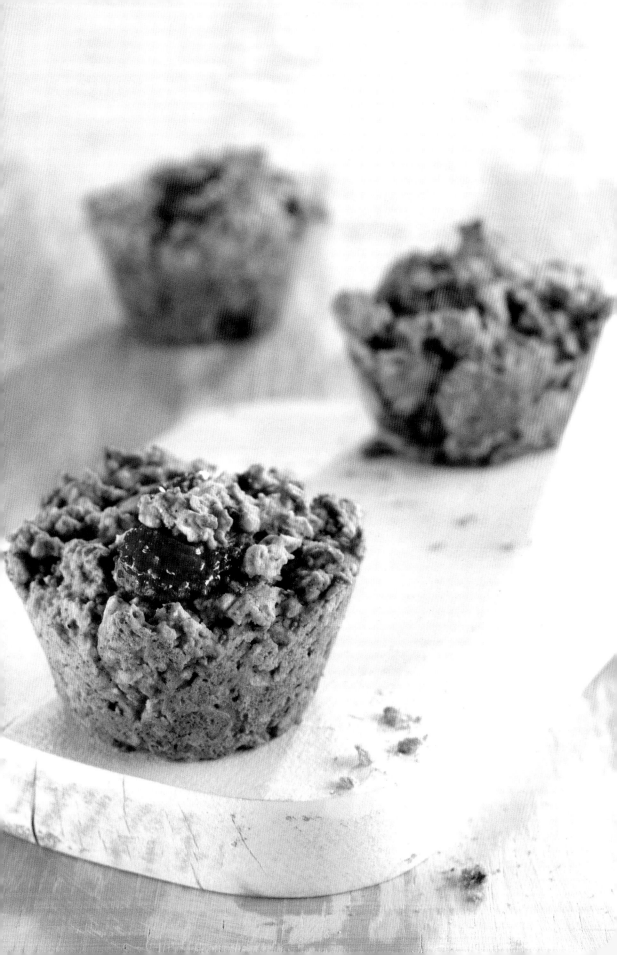

BANANA AND ALMOND
Butter Cookies

12 cookies • PREPARATION: 10 minutes • COOKING TIME: 12 minutes

INGREDIENTS

1 very ripe banana

¼ cup (60 ml) natural almond butter
or peanut butter

1 egg

¼ cup (60 ml) brown sugar

½ cup (125 ml) lactose-free milk
or plain soy milk

1¼ cups (300 ml) gluten-free pastry
flour mix

1 tsp baking powder

METHOD

Preheat oven to 350°F (180°C). Line a baking sheet with parchment paper.

In a bowl, using a fork, mash banana. Add almond or peanut butter, egg, brown sugar and milk.

Whisk together to blend thoroughly.

In another bowl, combine flour and baking powder. Pour wet mixture into dry mixture and blend thoroughly.

On prepared baking sheet, drop 2 tbsp of dough per cookie to form 12 cookies. Press down lightly with the back of a spoon.

Bake in preheated oven for 12 minutes. Let cool on a rack.

Nutrition Facts
Per cookie

Amount	
Calories	114
Fat	4 g
Sodium	12 mg
Carbohydrates	17 g
Fiber	1 g
Protein	4 g

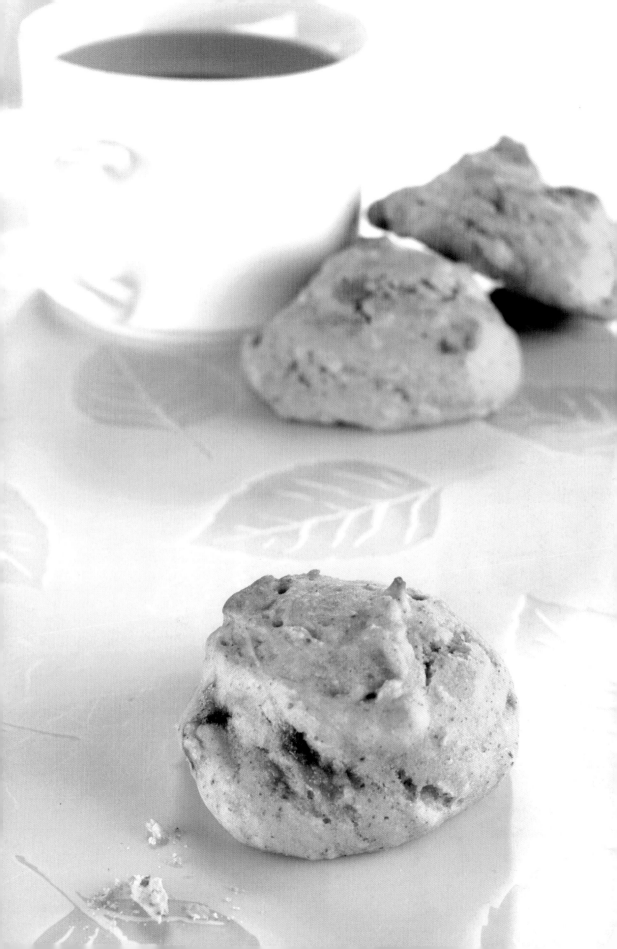

GRANOLA
with Dried Banana Chips

23 servings of ¼ cup (60 ml) • PREPARATION: 10 minutes • COOKING TIME: 20 minutes

INGREDIENTS

3 cups (750 ml) old-fashioned rolled oats

1 cup (250 ml) oat bran

2 tbsp maple syrup

2 eggs

1½ cups (375 ml) unsweetened dried banana chips

METHOD

Position rack in center of oven and preheat to 320°F (160°C).

In a bowl, combine rolled oats, oat bran, maple syrup and eggs.

Spread mixture on a baking sheet. Bake on middle rack in preheated oven for 15 to 20 minutes, stirring every 5 minutes, until granola is golden brown.

Let cool completely before adding banana chips.

• • • • • • • • • • • • •

TIP

Granola keeps at room temperature for up to 7 days or in the refrigerator for 2 weeks.

Nutrition Facts Per ¼ cup (60 ml) serving	
Amount	
Calories	100
Fat	4 g
Sodium	8 mg
Carbohydrates	16 g
Fiber	2 g
Protein	3 g

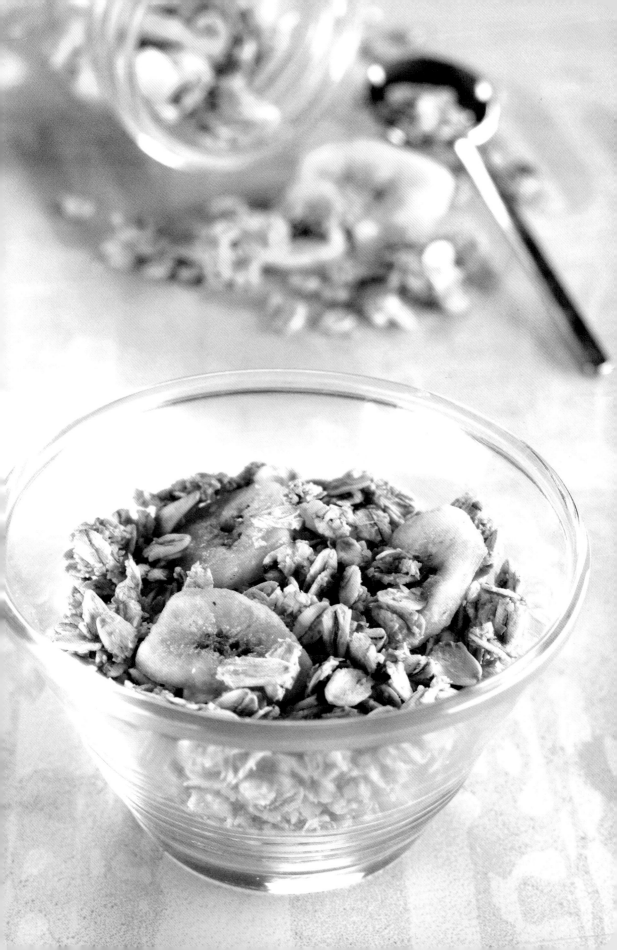

SALMON MOUSSE
Sandwiches

2 sandwiches • PREPARATION: 5 minutes

INGREDIENTS

1 can (7½ oz/213 g) boneless salmon, drained

2 tbsp lactose-free plain yogurt

1 tsp Dijon mustard

4 slices gluten-free bread

4 or 5 baby lettuce leaves

A few slices of tomato

For the seasonings

1 tbsp paprika

Salt and black pepper

METHOD

In a food processor or with a hand mixer, blend together salmon, yogurt, mustard and seasonings into a mousse.

Spread slices of bread with salmon mousse. Garnish with lettuce and tomato slices, then close sandwiches.

Serve with 2 cups (500 ml) low-FODMAP raw vegetables (see p. 20).

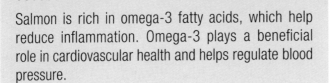

DIGESTIVE HEALTH INFO

Salmon is rich in omega-3 fatty acids, which help reduce inflammation. Omega-3 plays a beneficial role in cardiovascular health and helps regulate blood pressure.

Nutrition Facts Per sandwich	
Amount	
Calories	410
Fat	10 g
Sodium	700 mg
Carbohydrates	50 g
Fiber	4 g
Protein	27 g

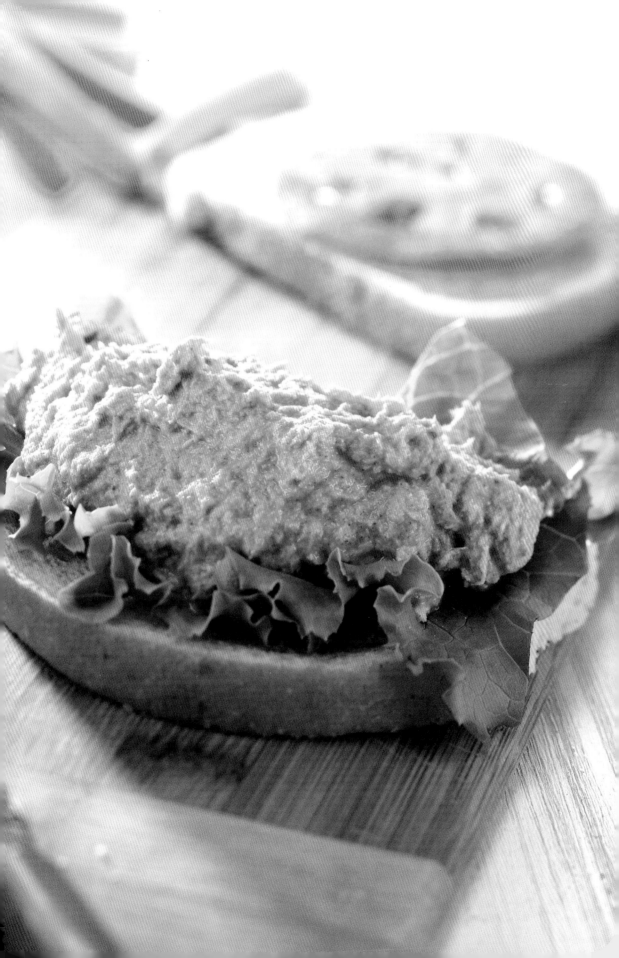

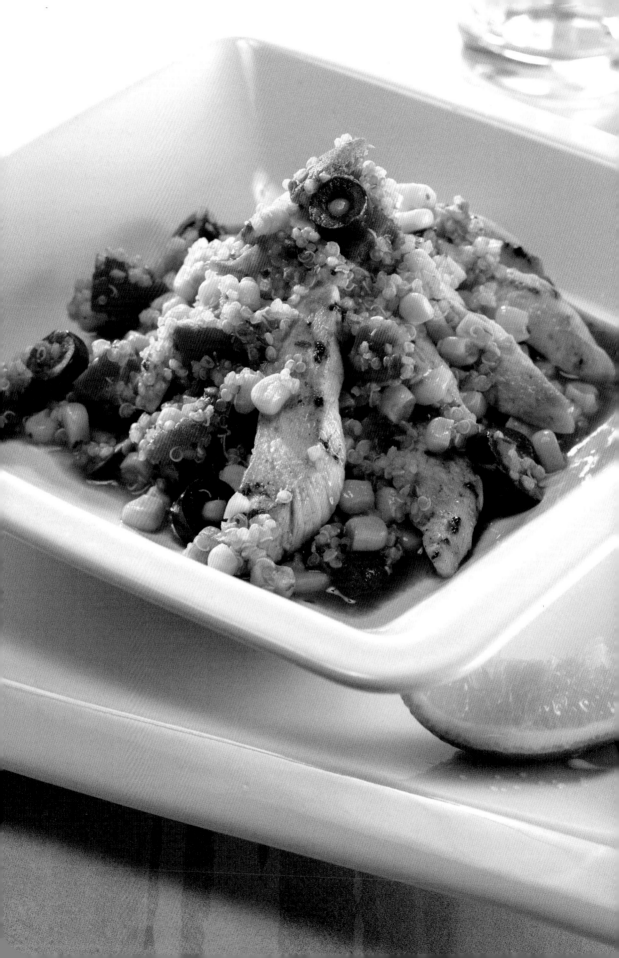

MEXICAN QUINOA
Salad

4 servings • PREPARATION: 15 minutes • COOKING TIME: 20 minutes

METHOD

In a saucepan, combine quinoa, 2 cups (500 ml) water and chicken bouillon powder and bring to a boil. Reduce heat to low and cook for 20 minutes.

Meanwhile, in a skillet, heat oil over medium heat. Add chicken, parsley, basil and pepper and cook, stirring frequently until browned, about 4 to 5 minutes.

In the saucepan containing quinoa, add seasoned chicken, tomatoes, corn and olives. Cook over low heat for 4 to 5 minutes, until chicken is no longer pink inside. Add lime juice and cilantro

INGREDIENTS

¾ cup (180 ml) quinoa, rinsed and drained

2 tsp chicken bouillon powder

1 tbsp olive oil

3 small boneless, skinless chicken breasts (about 14 oz/390 g), cut into strips

1 can (28 oz/796 ml) sodium-free diced tomatoes, half-drained

1 can (12 oz/341 ml) corn, drained

1 cup (250 ml) pitted black or green olives, sliced

1 tbsp lime juice

For the seasonings

1 tbsp dried parsley

1 tbsp dried basil

A few leaves fresh cilantro

Black pepper

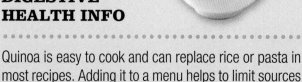

DIGESTIVE HEALTH INFO

Quinoa is easy to cook and can replace rice or pasta in most recipes. Adding it to a menu helps to limit sources of wheat and increase the variety of nutrients.

Nutrition Facts Per serving	
Amount	
Calories	459
Fat	13 g
Sodium	600 mg
Carbohydrates	54 g
Fiber	9 g
Protein	40 g

BELL PEPPER
Quiche

4 servings • PREPARATION: 15 minutes • COOKING TIME: 30 minutes

INGREDIENTS

1 tbsp canola oil	
2 stalks celery, chopped	
1 yellow bell pepper, julienned	
1 red bell pepper, julienned	
4 eggs	
1 cup (250 ml) lactose-free milk or plain soy milk	
1 cup (250 ml) grated Cheddar cheese	
¾ cup (180 ml) gluten-free flour	

For the seasonings

1 tbsp dried parsley	
1 tbsp dried basil	
1 tbsp fresh or dried chives	
Salt and black pepper	

METHOD

Preheat oven to 375°F (190°C). Lightly oil an 11-inch (28 cm) pie plate.

In a preheated skillet, heat oil over medium heat. Add celery and bell peppers and gently fry for 2 to 3 minutes. Set aside.

In a large bowl, using a fork, beat eggs with milk. Add cheese and flour, then vegetables and seasonings. Stir until evenly mixed.

Transfer mixture to prepared pie plate and bake in preheated oven for 30 minutes.

Serve with a salad of low-FODMAP vegetables (see p. 20).

• • • • • • • • • • • • • •

TIP

This recipe can be precooked in a microwave on maximum power for 3 minutes, covered, or 2 minutes, uncovered. Finish cooking in a preheated oven at 375°F (190°C) for 10 minutes.

Nutrition Facts
Per serving

Amount	
Calories	367
Fat	20 g
Sodium	290 mg
Carbohydrates	26 g
Fiber	2 g
Protein	20 g

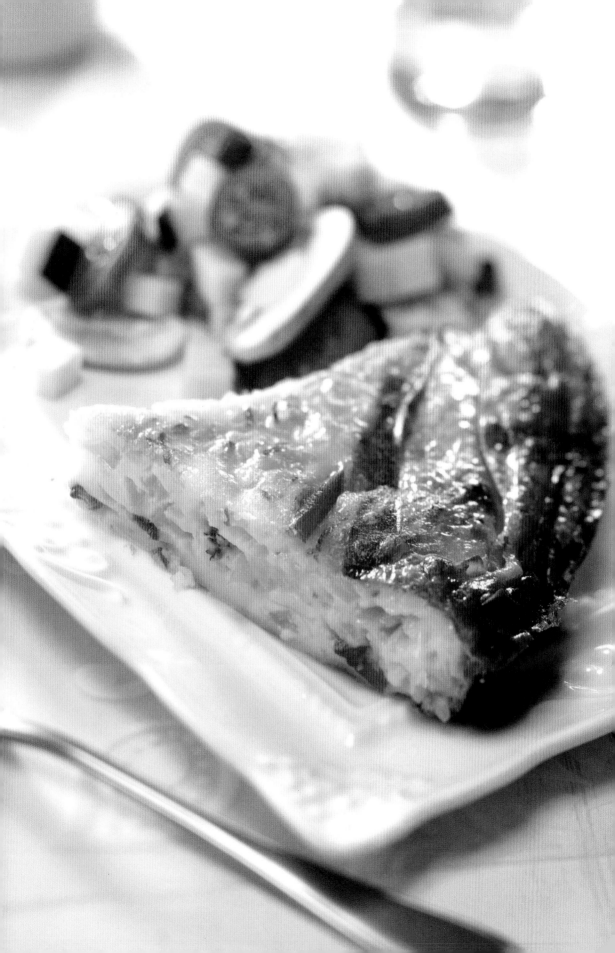

HERBED SOLE
Casserole

4 servings • PREPARATION: 20 minutes • COOKING TIME: 20 minutes

INGREDIENTS

1 tbsp canola oil

2 stalks celery, chopped

3 cups (750 ml) low-sodium chicken broth

2 tbsp Dijon mustard

1 cup (250 ml) millet

4 large fillets of sole (1 lb/500 g)

2 red bell peppers, diced

4 cups (1 liter) green beans, cut in pieces

For the seasonings

2 tbsp dried thyme

2 tbsp dried parsley

1 tbsp dried oregano

Salt and black pepper

METHOD

In a saucepan, heat oil over medium heat. Add celery and gently fry for a few minutes. Add broth, mustard and seasonings, then bring to a boil. Add millet and cook for 15 minutes.

Add fish, bell peppers and green beans. Reduce heat to low. Cover and cook for 5 minutes.

• • • • • • • • • • • • • •

VARIATION

Replace sole with another white fish like tilapia or cod.

Nutrition Facts	
Per serving	
Amount	
Calories	426
Fat	8 g
Sodium	655 mg
Carbohydrates	52 g
Fiber	9 g
Protein	35 g

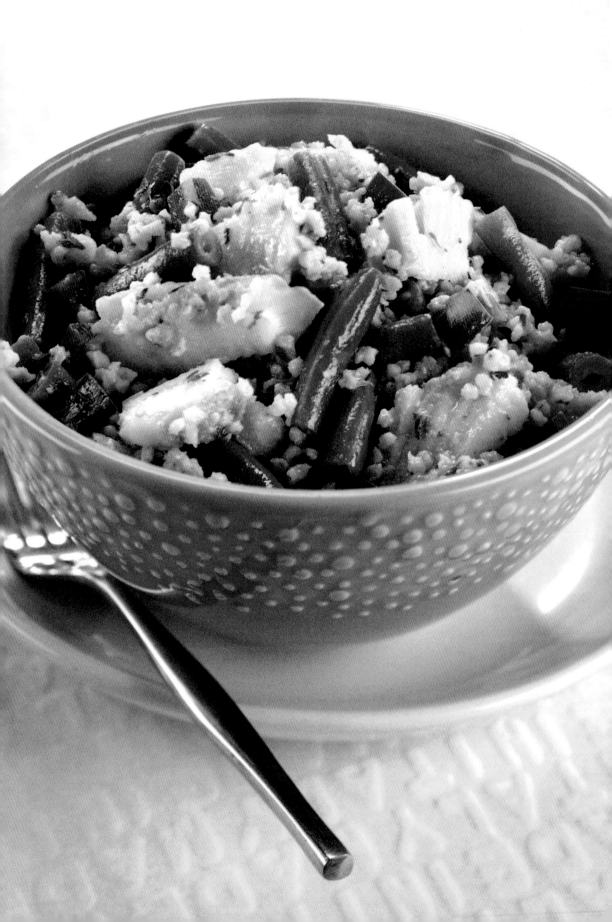

BEEF AND RICE
Soup

5 servings • PREPARATION: 20 minutes • COOKING TIME: 25 minutes

INGREDIENTS

1 lb (500 g) beef, cut into small cubes

2 tbsp gluten-free flour

2 tbsp canola oil

2 stalks celery, chopped

3 carrots, cut into chunks

2 tbsp beef bouillon powder

1 cup (250 ml) green beans,
cut in pieces

½ cup (125 ml) brown rice

1 can (28 oz/796 ml) crushed
tomatoes

METHOD

Coat beef cubes in flour.

In a saucepan, heat oil over medium heat. Add celery and carrots and gently fry for a few minutes. Add beef cubes and gently fry for 2 minutes.

Dilute beef bouillon powder in 6 cups (1.5 liters) boiling water, then pour into saucepan. Add green beans and rice. Bring to a boil. Reduce heat and simmer for 20 minutes.

Add crushed tomatoes and continue cooking for 5 minutes.

• • • • • • • • • • • • • •

TIP

This soup is easy to freeze. It's a good way to prepare meals ahead of time.

Nutrition Facts	
Per serving	
Amount	
Calories	350
Fat	13 g
Sodium	444 mg
Carbohydrates	35 g
Fiber	6 g
Protein	25 g

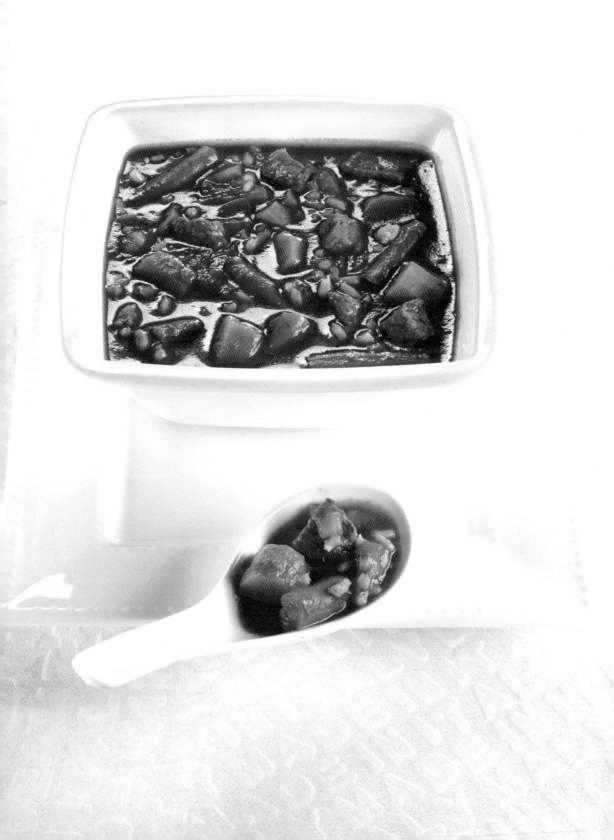

PORK STUFFED
with Olives

6 servings • PREPARATION: 30 minutes • COOKING TIME: 15 minutes

INGREDIENTS

13 oz (375 g) gluten-free fettuccini

1 cup (250 ml) shredded mozzarella cheese

¾ cup (180 ml) canned pitted black olives, sliced

1 large stalk celery, finely chopped

2 small pork tenderloins (about 14 oz/390 g)

2 tbsp olive oil

2 zucchini, cut into pieces

2 cups (500 ml) cherry tomatoes, cut in half

For the seasonings

1 tbsp dried basil

Salt and black pepper

METHOD

In a large pot of boiling water, cook pasta according to directions on package.

In a bowl, combine cheese, olives, celery and seasonings.

Cut pork tenderloins lengthwise without completely separating the two pieces. Spread cheese and olive mixture inside the tenderloins. Close tenderloins and tie with butcher's twine.

In a lightly oiled skillet over medium heat, cook tenderloins for 5 to 6 minutes on each side.

In another skillet, heat oil over medium heat. Add zucchini and cherry tomatoes and gently fry for 2 to 3 minutes. Add pasta.

Slice pork tenderloins and serve with pasta and vegetables.

Nutrition Facts
Per serving

Amount	
Calories	410
Fat	13 g
Sodium	478 mg
Carbohydrates	46 g
Fiber	7 g
Protein	29 g

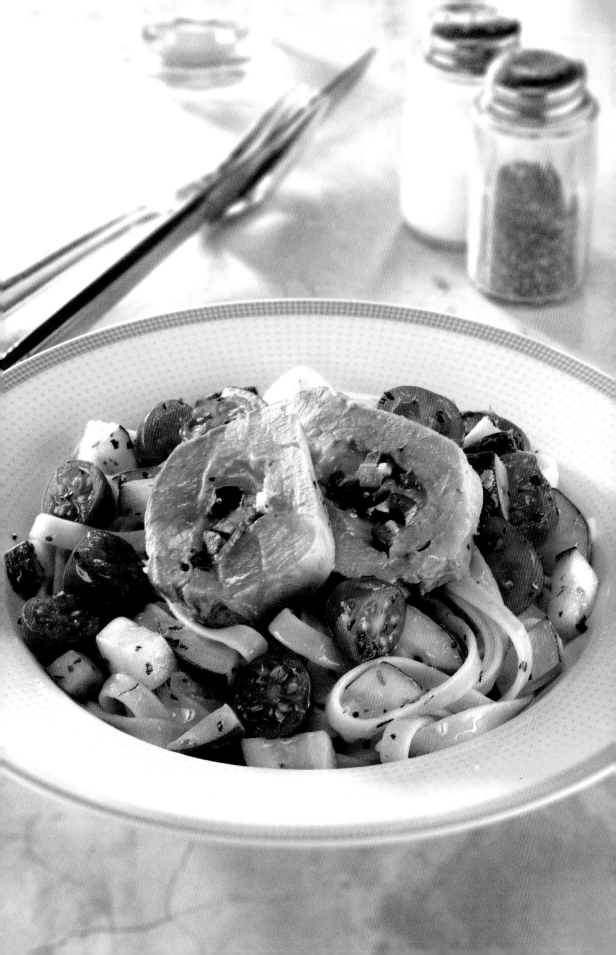

PINEAPPLE
Chicken

4 servings • PREPARATION: 20 minutes • COOKING TIME: 20 minutes

INGREDIENTS

¾ cup (180 ml) long-grain brown rice

4 small boneless, skinless chicken breasts (about 14 oz/390 g)

4 cups (1 liter) diced pineapple

2 cups (500 ml) green beans, cut in pieces

2 medium-size carrots, cut in small pieces

For the seasonings

1 tbsp dried thyme

Salt and black pepper

METHOD

Preheat oven to 350°F (180°C).

In a saucepan, cook rice according to directions on package.

Meanwhile, in a square baking dish, place chicken, pineapple, green beans, carrots and seasonings. Bake in preheated oven for 20 minutes or until chicken is no longer pink inside.

Serve chicken with rice.

Nutrition Facts Per serving	
Amount	
Calories	402
Fat	3 g
Sodium	108 mg
Carbohydrates	67 g
Fiber	7 g
Protein	28 g

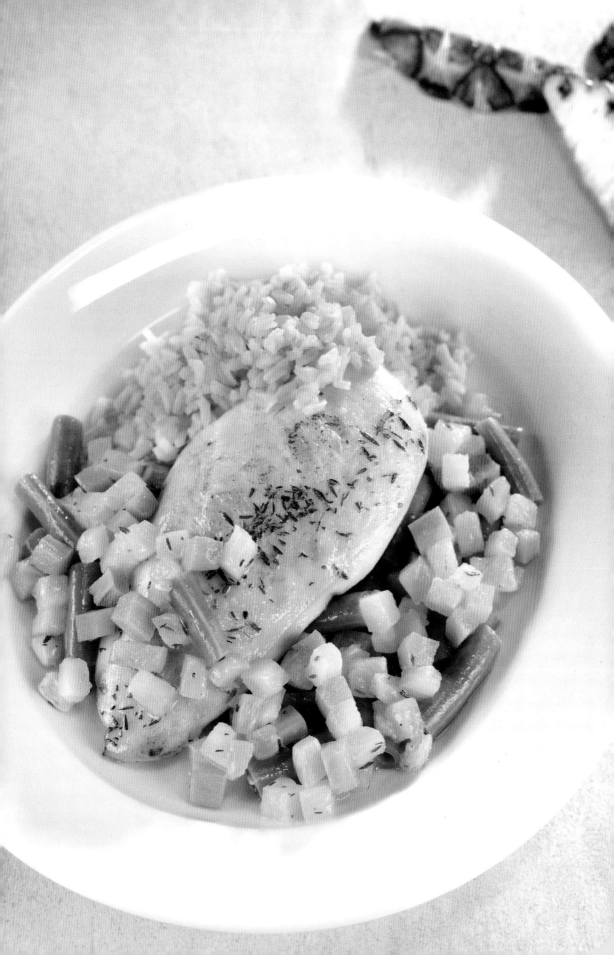

EASY
Stew

6 servings • PREPARATION: 20 minutes • COOKING TIME: 30 minutes

INGREDIENTS

1 lb (500 g) lean ground beef

3 tbsp cornstarch

2 tbsp beef bouillon powder

2 stalks celery, chopped

4 carrots, diced

1 cup (250 ml) diced turnip

4 potatoes, diced

For the seasonings

2 tbsp dried thyme

1 tbsp dried oregano

Black pepper

METHOD

Using your hands, form ground beef into 12 meatballs. Press firmly to prevent them from falling apart during cooking.

In a large saucepan, dissolve cornstarch and beef bouillon powder in 4 cups (1 liter) boiling water.

Add remaining ingredients including meatballs and stir gently. Cover and bring to a boil. Reduce heat to low and simmer for 25 to 30 minutes or until meatballs are no longer pink inside.

Nutrition Facts Per serving	
Amount	
Calories	271
Fat	11 g
Sodium	166 mg
Carbohydrates	22 g
Fiber	3 g
Protein	19 g

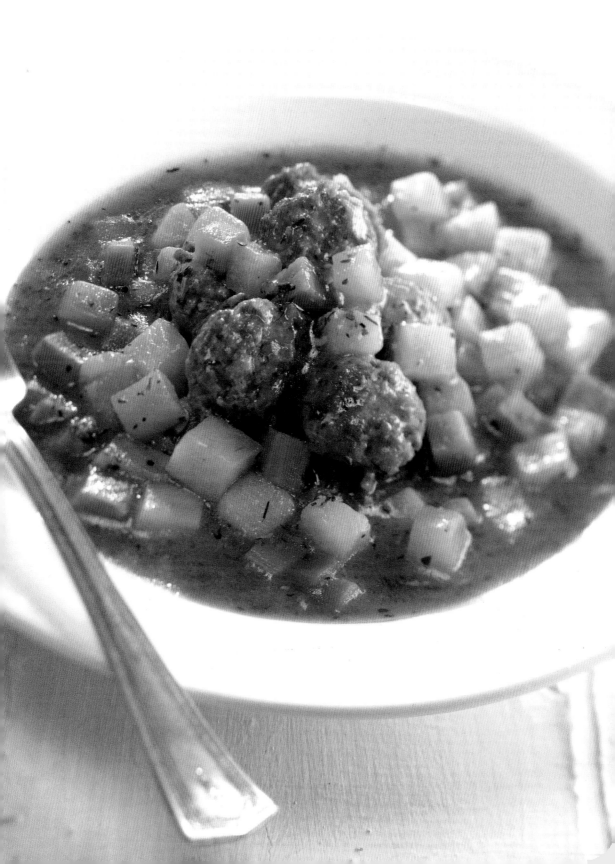

EGG
Tacos

4 servings • PREPARATION: 15 minutes • COOKING TIME: 5 minutes

INGREDIENTS

8 eggs

½ cup (125 ml) lactose-free milk or water

6 to 8 gluten-free tacos

2 red bell peppers, cut into strips

½ cup (125 ml) grated Swiss cheese

1 cup (250 ml) coarsely torn lettuce leaves

For the seasonings

1 tbsp chili powder

1 tsp Cajun seasoning

1 tsp paprika

Salt and black pepper

METHOD

In a bowl, beat eggs with milk and seasonings.

In a lightly oiled skillet over low heat, cook egg mixture, stirring constantly with a spatula, for about 5 minutes.

Fill tacos with egg mixture, bell peppers, cheese and lettuce.

• • • • • • • • • • • • • •

VARIATION

If you are particularly sensitive to stronger seasonings, it is recommended that you replace the chili and Cajun seasonings with milder herbs such as dried basil and thyme.

Nutrition Facts Per serving	
Amount	
Calories	325
Fat	20 g
Sodium	310 mg
Carbohydrates	17 g
Fiber	2 g
Protein	18 g

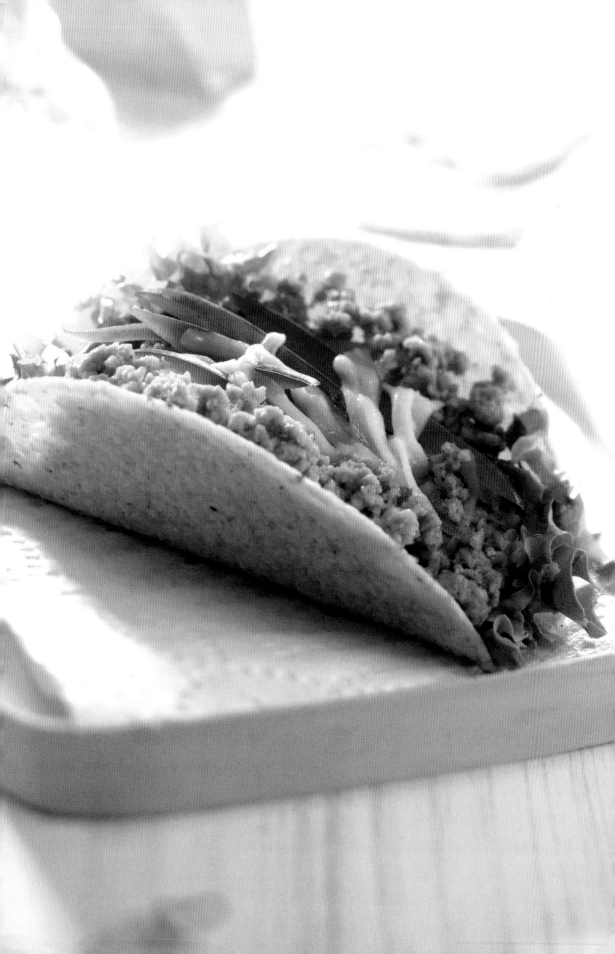

SIMMERED
Chicken

4 servings • PREPARATION: 15 minutes • COOKING TIME: 25 minutes

INGREDIENTS

2 tbsp canola oil

2 stalks celery, chopped

2 large boneless, skinless chicken breasts (about 14 oz/390 g), cut into cubes

2 tbsp gluten-free flour

2 tbsp chicken bouillon powder

½ cup (125 ml) long-grain brown rice

2 cups (500 ml) diced butternut squash

2 sweet potatoes, diced (2 cups/500 ml)

For the seasonings

2 bay leaves

1 tbsp dried thyme

1 tbsp dried rosemary

1 tbsp dried tarragon

Black pepper

METHOD

In a saucepan, heat oil over medium heat. Add celery and gently fry for a few minutes.

Coat chicken cubes in flour. Add to celery in saucepan and gently fry for 2 minutes. Add 4 cups (1 liter) water, chicken bouillon powder dissolved in a bit of boiling water, rice and seasonings. Cook over low heat for 15 minutes.

Add squash and sweet potatoes and continue cooking for 10 minutes until vegetables are tender and chicken is no longer pink inside.

• • • • • • • • • • • • • •

TIP

To avoid any contamination, it is essential to wash your hands as well as the utensils you have used after handling raw chicken, especially the cutting board you use, whether plastic or wood.

Nutrition Facts	
Per serving	
Amount	
Calories	361
Fat	10 g
Sodium	245 mg
Carbohydrates	40 g
Fiber	4 g
Protein	28 g

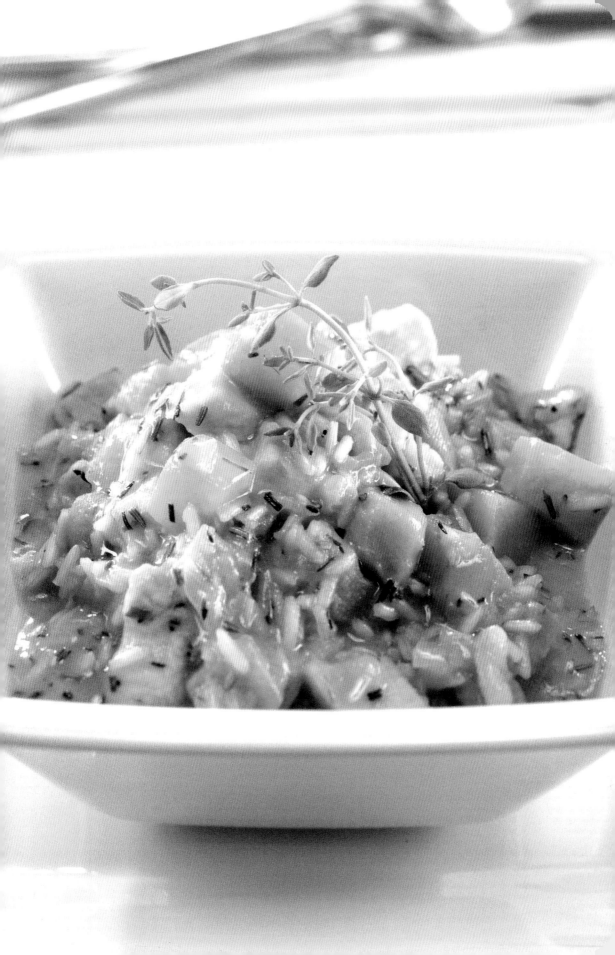

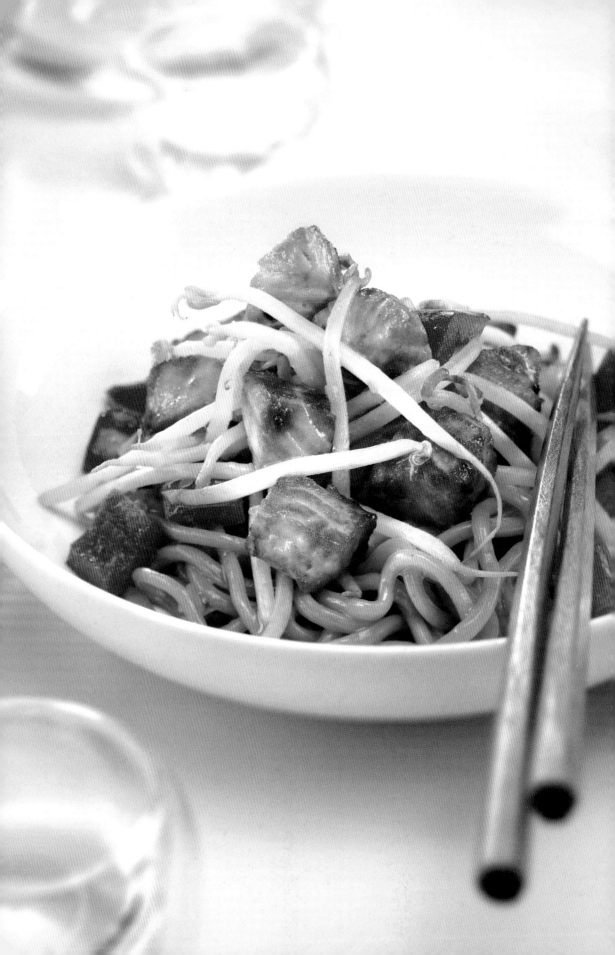

4 servings • PREPARATION: 20 minutes • REFRIGERATION: 20 minutes • COOKING TIME: 15 minutes

METHOD

In a bowl, combine soy sauce, maple syrup and rice vinegar. Add salmon cubes, mix together thoroughly and marinate for 20 minutes in the refrigerator.

Meanwhile, in a large pot of boiling water, cook noodles according to instructions on the package.

In a preheated skillet, heat oil over medium heat. Add celery and gently fry for a few minutes. Remove salmon cubes from marinade, reserving marinade. Gently fry salmon cubes in skillet for 1 minute on each side. Remove from skillet and set aside.

In same skillet, gently fry bell peppers and bean sprouts for 3 to 4 minutes. Add reserved marinade and salmon, stirring gently to avoid breaking up the fish. Cook for about 5 minutes.

Serve salmon with soba noodles.

INGREDIENTS

2 tbsp low-sodium soy sauce

1 tbsp maple syrup

1 tbsp rice vinegar

2 salmon fillets, skin removed, cut into cubes

4 oz (120 g) gluten-free soba noodles, gluten-free pasta or rice vermicelli

1 tbsp sesame or canola oil

2 stalks celery, chopped

3 red bell peppers, cut into pieces

4 cups (1 liter) bean sprouts

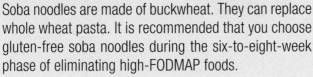

DIGESTIVE HEALTH INFO

Soba noodles are made of buckwheat. They can replace whole wheat pasta. It is recommended that you choose gluten-free soba noodles during the six-to-eight-week phase of eliminating high-FODMAP foods.

Nutrition Facts	
Per serving	
Amount	
Calories	520
Fat	25 g
Sodium	645 mg
Carbohydrates	39 g
Fiber	2 g
Protein	40 g

MEAL SALAD

4 servings • PREPARATION: 15 minutes • COOKING TIME: 10 minutes

INGREDIENTS

4 cups (1 liter) gluten-free fresh pasta, ravioli or tortellini, with your choice of filling

2 cups (500 ml) cherry tomatoes

2 zucchini, diced

2 tbsp olive oil

Juice of 1 lemon

4 hard-boiled eggs, sliced or halved

For the seasonings

1 tbsp dried basil

Salt and black pepper

METHOD

In a large pot of boiling water, cook pasta according to directions on package.

Drain pasta, then add tomatoes, zucchini, oil, lemon and seasonings. Mix thoroughly, then top with eggs.

Serve salad warm or cold.

• • • • • • • • • • • • •

TIP

You can keep this salad up to 5 days in the refrigerator.

• • • • • • • • • • • • •

VARIATION

Choose different vegetables to vary this recipe: baby spinach leaves, cooked green beans, etc.

Nutrition Facts Per serving	
Amount	
Calories	390
Fat	14 g
Sodium	88 mg
Carbohydrates	50 g
Fiber	4 g
Protein	17 g

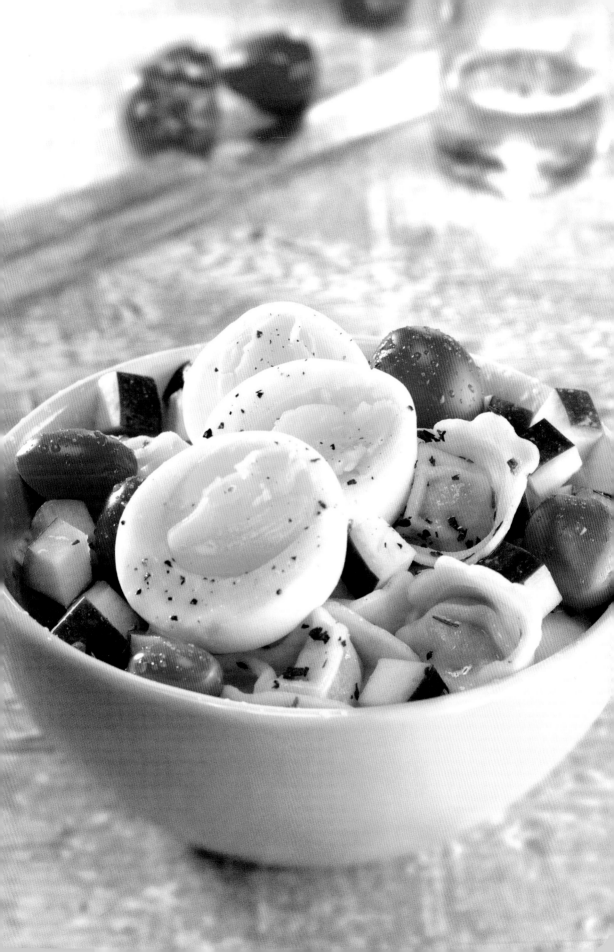

VEGETARIAN
Casserole

5 servings • PREPARATION: 15 minutes • REFRIGERATION: 15 minutes to 2 hours •
COOKING TIME: 40 minutes

INGREDIENTS

2 tbsp low-sodium soy sauce

2 tbsp olive oil

Juice of 2 limes

1 lb 5 oz (650 g) firm tofu,
cut into large cubes

2 tomatoes, diced

2 zucchini, diced

1 red bell pepper, diced

2 tbsp cornstarch

2 cups (500 ml) grated Cheddar
cheese

For the seasonings

1 tbsp dried thyme

1 tbsp dried basil

Black pepper

METHOD

Preheat oven to 350°F (180°C).

In a bowl, combine soy sauce, oil, lime juice, 2 tbsp water and seasonings. Add tofu and marinate for at least 15 minutes or for up to 2 hours in the refrigerator.

Drain tofu and set aside marinade. In a baking dish, spread out pieces of tofu. Add tomatoes, zucchini and bell pepper.

Dilute cornstarch in reserved marinade. Pour over tofu and vegetables. Top with cheese and bake in preheated oven for 30 to 45 minutes until cheese is bubbling and vegetables are tender.

Serve with quinoa or rice.

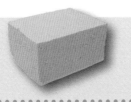

DIGESTIVE HEALTH INFO

Tofu is a plant protein. It is lower in fat than meat and easy to digest. Some people, however, may have more bloating and gas after eating soy-based products.

Nutrition Facts	
Per serving	
Amount	
Calories	338
Fat	23 g
Sodium	628 mg
Carbohydrates	18 g
Fiber	3 g
Protein	33 g

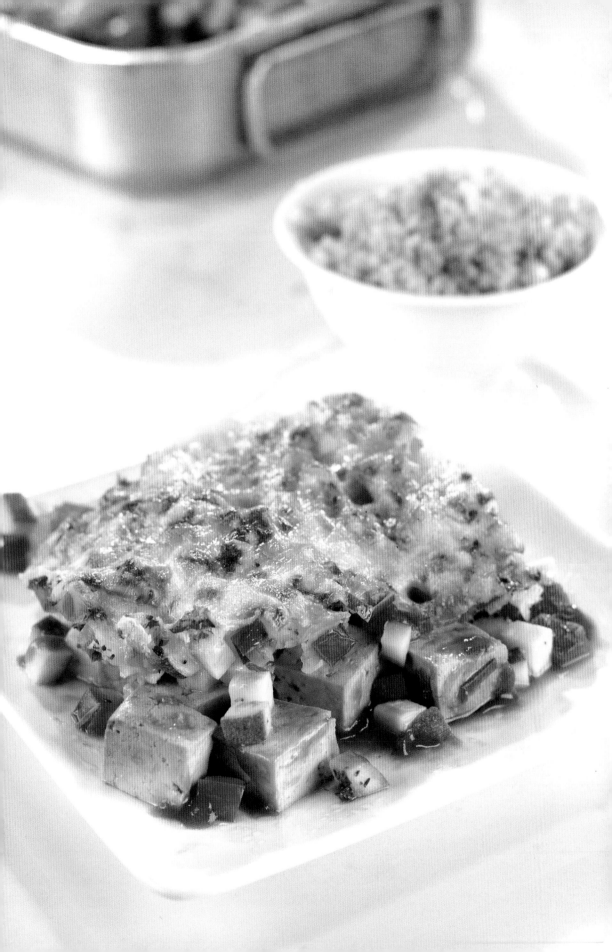

SHRIMP
Brochettes

4 servings • PREPARATION: 20 minutes • REFRIGERATION: 10 minutes • COOKING TIME: 10 minutes

INGREDIENTS

1 cup (250 ml) jasmine or other rice

2 tbsp olive oil

16 large uncooked, deveined shrimp

2 yellow or red bell peppers,
cut into pieces

1 cup (250 ml) cubed pineapple

2 lemons, quartered

For the seasonings

1 tbsp dried thyme

1 tbsp chopped fresh chives

Salt and black pepper

METHOD

Preheat oven to 350°F (180°C).

In a saucepan, cook rice according to directions on package.

Meanwhile, in a bowl, combine oil and seasonings. Add shrimp, mix together and marinate for 10 minutes in the refrigerator.

Assemble brochettes, alternating shrimp, bell pepper pieces, pineapple cubes and lemon wedges. Place on a grill plate or baking sheet and cook in preheated oven for 2 minutes. Turn brochettes and continue cooking for 2 minutes more.

Serve brochettes with rice.

• • • • • • • • • • • • • •

TIP

Cook a large quantity of rice and freeze in individual servings to always have on hand.

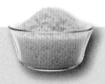

DIGESTIVE HEALTH INFO

Rice is one of the least allergenic grains. It is recommended that you choose long-grain rice over instant rice, which contains little fiber and is not very nourishing. Choose a type of rice that contains at least 2 grams of fiber per ½ cup (125 ml) of uncooked rice.

Nutrition Facts Per serving	
Amount	
Calories	350
Fat	9 g
Sodium	500 mg
Carbohydrates	50 g
Fiber	3 g
Protein	19 g

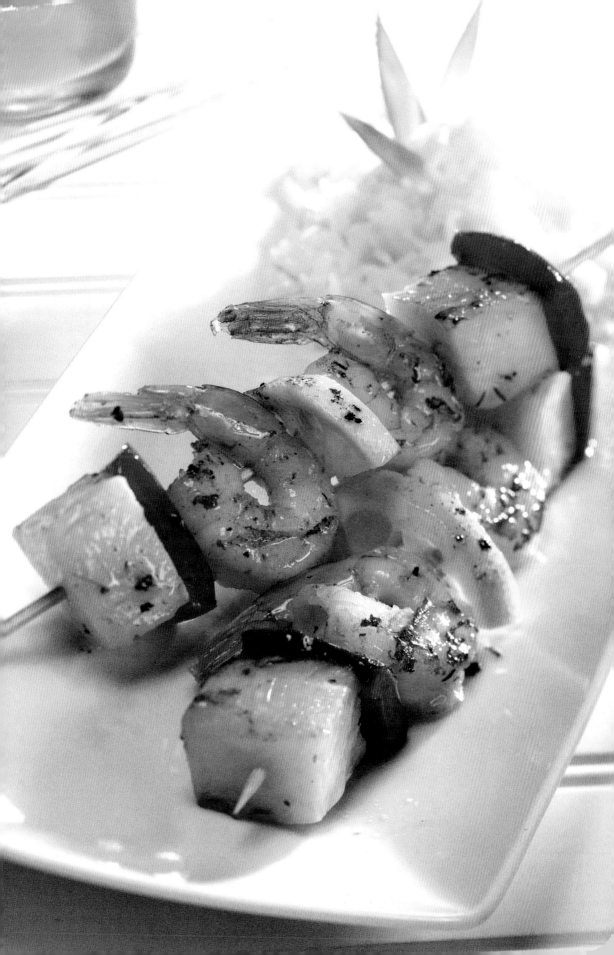

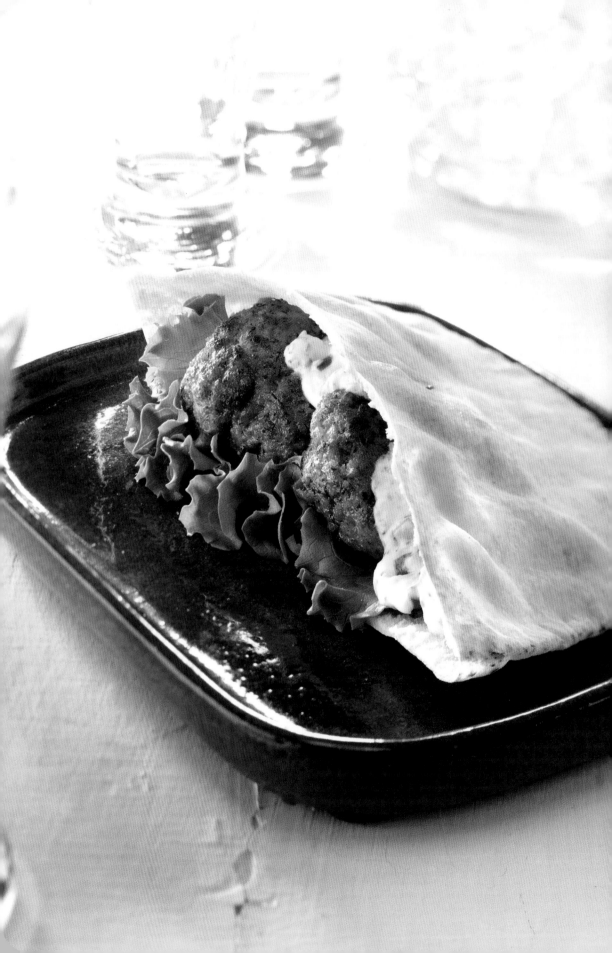

VEAL PITA POCKETS
with Tzatziki

6 servings • PREPARATION: 20 minutes • COOKING TIME: 15 minutes

METHOD

In a bowl, combine yogurt, cucumber and dill. Add salt and black pepper to taste. Let sit until ready to serve.

In a large bowl, combine ground veal, breadcrumbs, mustard and basil. Add salt and black pepper to taste.

Using your hands, form 12 small croquettes and flatten to the diameter of the bottom of a glass.

In a skillet, heat oil over medium heat. Add croquettes and cook, turning frequently, about 12 minutes.

Cut pitas in half. Place 2 croquettes inside each pita half. Fill with yogurt sauce and lettuce leaves.

• • • • • • • • • • • • • •

TIP

Prepare a large quantity of veal croquettes and freeze them in a resealable airtight bag. This will allow you to have quick meals on hand any time

INGREDIENTS

1 cup (250 ml) lactose-free plain yogurt or low-fat sour cream

1 cup (250 ml) peeled, finely diced cucumber

1 lb (500 g) ground veal

½ cup (125 ml) gluten-free breadcrumbs

1 tbsp Dijon mustard

1 tbsp canola oil

3 medium-size gluten-free pitas

A few leaves Boston lettuce

For the seasonings

1 tbsp dried dill

1 tbsp dried basil

Salt and black pepper

Nutrition Facts	
Per serving	
Amount	
Calories	315
Fat	10 g
Sodium	420 mg
Carbohydrates	34 g
Fiber	4 g
Protein	23 g

CHINESE-STYLE
Pork and Rice

4 servings • PREPARATION: 15 minutes • COOKING TIME: 20 minutes

INGREDIENTS

1 cup (250 ml) long-grain brown rice

1 tbsp canola oil

2 stalks celery, chopped

14 oz (390 g) small boneless pork chops, cut into strips

2 tbsp low-sodium soy sauce

1 tbsp brown sugar

2 red bell peppers, diced

2 cups (500 ml) bean sprouts

For the seasonings

1 tbsp fresh or dried basil

Salt and black pepper

METHOD

In a saucepan, cook rice according to directions on package.

About 10 minutes before rice is cooked, in a large skillet, heat oil over medium-low heat. Add celery and gently fry for a few minutes. Add pork and cook over low heat for 5 to 6 minutes.

Add soy sauce, brown sugar, bell peppers, bean sprouts and seasonings. Continue to cook for 3 to 4 minutes.

Add rice and mix thoroughly.

Nutrition Facts
Per serving

Amount	
Calories	423
Fat	11 g
Sodium	385 mg
Carbohydrates	50 g
Fiber	4 g
Protein	32 g

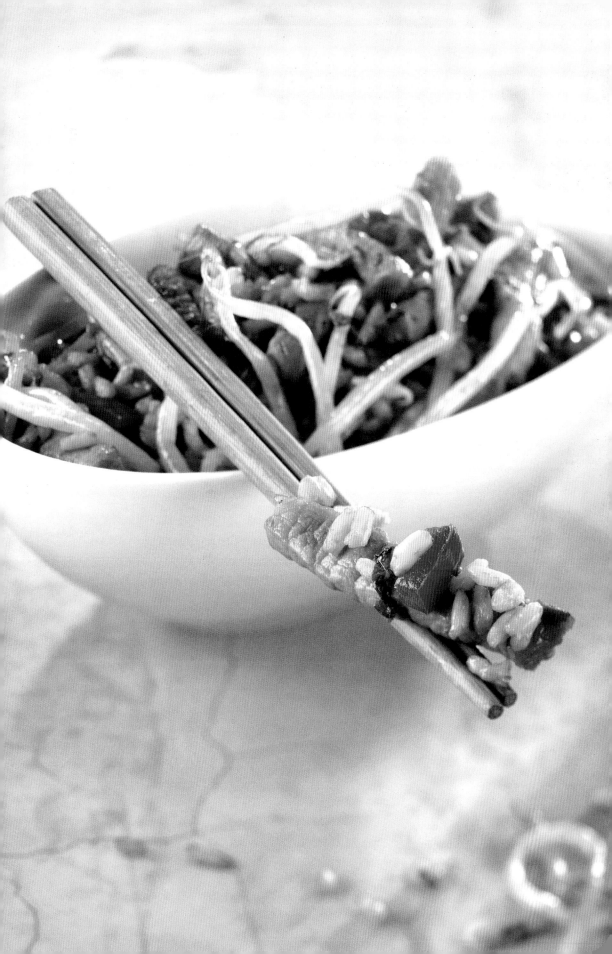

ASIAN
Soup

5 to 6 servings • PREPARATION: 15 minutes • REFRIGERATION: 20 minutes • COOKING TIME: 15 minutes

INGREDIENTS

2 tbsp low-sodium soy sauce

2 tbsp fresh grated ginger

2 tsp lime juice

10 oz (300 g) firm silken tofu, diced

2 stalks celery, chopped

1 tbsp sesame oil

3 cups (750 ml) low-sodium chicken broth

1 can (14 oz/398 ml) coconut milk

1 red bell pepper, julienned

1 carrot, thinly sliced

1 cup (250 ml) bean sprouts

4 oz (120 g) rice vermicelli

METHOD

In a bowl, combine soy sauce, ginger and lime juice. Add tofu and marinate for at least 20 minutes in the refrigerator.

In a saucepan, heat oil over medium heat. Add celery and gently fry for a few minutes. Add chicken broth and coconut milk. Add tofu, marinade, bell pepper, carrot and bean sprouts. Simmer over low heat for 6 to 7 minutes.

Meanwhile, place rice vermicelli in a large bowl and add 4 cups (1 liter) boiling water. Let sit for 5 minutes, then drain.

Distribute rice vermicelli into individual bowls and pour soup on top.

Nutrition Facts
Per serving
($^1/_6$ of recipe)

Amount	
Calories	310
Fat	20 g
Sodium	424 mg
Carbohydrates	24 g
Fiber	2 g
Protein	10 g

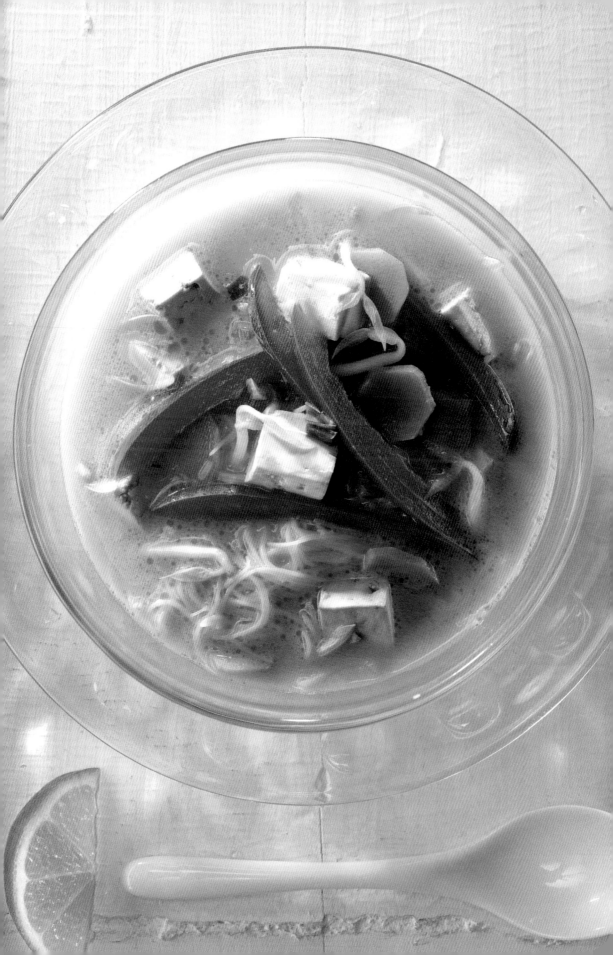

CHEESE
Cannelloni

4 to 6 servings • PREPARATION: 20 minutes • COOKING TIME: 40 minutes

INGREDIENTS

3 tbsp olive oil

2 stalks celery, chopped

1 cup (250 ml) cooked spinach, drained and chopped

1 egg, beaten

1½ cups (375 ml) grated Gruyère cheese

1 cup (250 ml) grated Swiss cheese, divided

12 gluten-free cannelloni pasta

3 cups (750 ml) tomato sauce

For the seasonings

1 tbsp dried basil

1 tbsp dried thyme

1 tbsp dried parsley

Salt and black pepper

METHOD

Preheat oven to 350°F (180°C).

In a preheated skillet, heat oil over medium heat. Add celery and gently fry for a few minutes. Transfer to a large bowl. Add spinach, egg, Gruyère cheese, ½ cup (125 ml) of the Swiss cheese and seasonings.

Fill cannelloni with spinach mixture. Place in a large baking dish. Combine tomato sauce with 1 cup (250 ml) water and add to baking dish. Top with remaining grated Swiss cheese. Bake in preheated oven for 30 to 40 minutes or according to directions on package of cannelloni.

Serve with a salad of low-FODMAP vegetables (see p. 20).

• • • • • • • • • • • • • •

TIP

To save time, cook cannelloni in boiling water until half cooked. Add only ½ cup (125 ml) of water to tomato sauce before placing dish in oven.

Nutrition Facts	
Per serving (1/6 of recipe)	
Amount	
Calories	462
Fat	24 g
Sodium	750 mg
Carbohydrates	40 g
Fiber	5 g
Protein	24 g

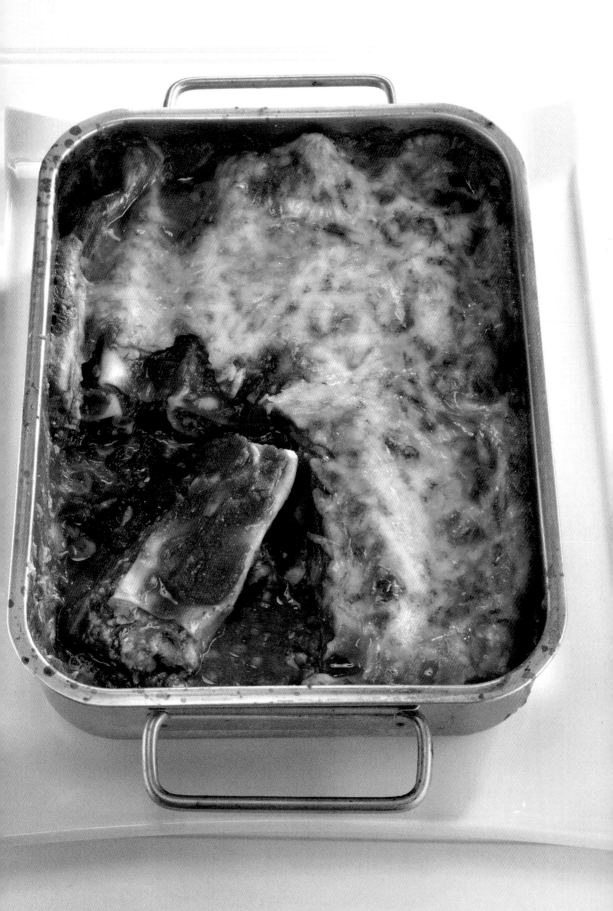

BREADED
Fish

4 servings • PREPARATION: 35 minutes • COOKING TIME: 15 minutes

INGREDIENTS

2 tbsp canola oil, divided

2 stalks celery, chopped

3 cups (750 ml) low-sodium chicken broth

¾ cup (180 ml) millet

1 cup (250 ml) gluten-free bread-crumbs

2 eggs, beaten

4 tilapia fillets (about 14 oz/390 g)

2 carrots, diced

1 cup (250 ml) green beans, cut in pieces

Juice of 1 lemon

For the seasonings

1 tbsp dried thyme

1 tbsp dried dill

Salt and black pepper

Nutrition Facts Per serving	
Amount	
Calories	489
Fat	14 g
Sodium	800 mg
Carbohydrates	56 g
Fiber	7 g
Protein	33 g

METHOD

In a saucepan, heat 1 tbsp of the oil over medium heat. Add celery and gently fry for a few minutes. Add chicken broth and millet. Bring to a boil. Reduce heat to low. Cover and simmer for 30 minutes.

Meanwhile, in a bowl, combine bread-crumbs and seasonings.

In another bowl, beat eggs. Dip tilapia fillets in beaten egg, then in seasoned breadcrumbs.

In a preheated skillet, heat remaining oil over medium heat. Add fillets and brown for 3 minutes. Gently turn fillets over and continue cooking for 3 minutes.

In a microwave-safe bowl, combine carrots and green beans in a small quantity of water and cook in microwave for 4 to 5 minutes until tender but still slightly crisp.

Drizzle fish with lemon juice and serve with vegetables and millet.

• • • • • • • • • • • • • •

VARIATIONS

• Replace tilapia with another white fish like sole or cod.

• Replace half the breadcrumbs with oat bran.

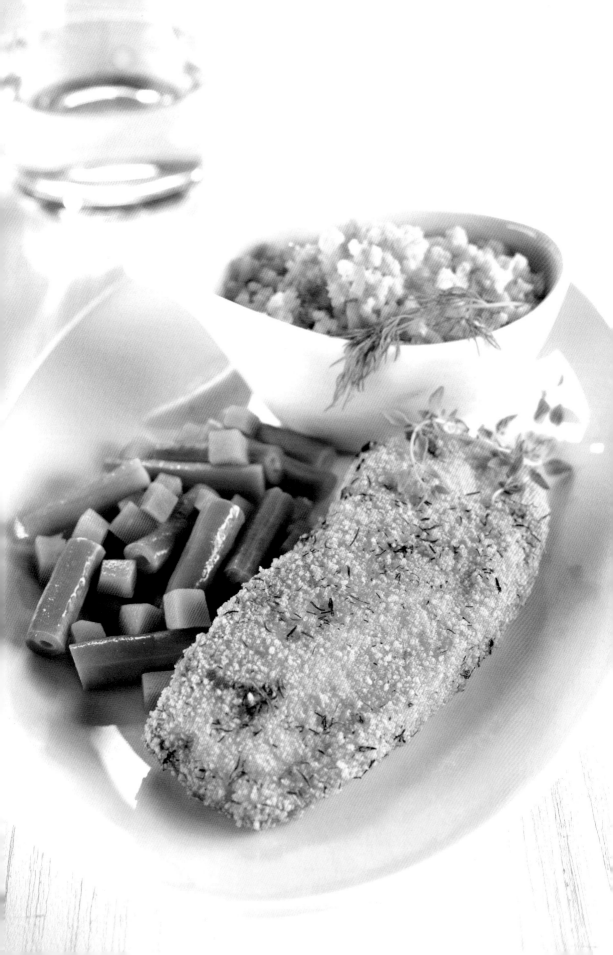

CHICKEN
in Peanut Sauce

4 servings • PREPARATION: 15 minutes • COOKING TIME: 15 minutes

INGREDIENTS

1 tbsp sesame oil

4 small boneless, skinless chicken breasts (about 14 oz/390 g), cut into pieces

4 oz (120 g) rice vermicelli

½ cup (125 ml) natural peanut butter

1 tbsp maple syrup

2 tbsp low-sodium soy sauce

2 red bell peppers, cut into pieces

3 cups (750 ml) bean sprouts

For the seasonings

Crushed red pepper flakes

Black pepper

METHOD

In a skillet, heat oil over medium heat. Add chicken pieces and gently fry for 5 to 6 minutes.

Meanwhile, in a bowl, combine rice vermicelli and 4 cups (1 liter) boiling water. Let sit for 5 minutes, then drain.

In a microwave-safe measuring cup, combine peanut butter, maple syrup, soy sauce, ½ cup (125 ml) water and seasonings. Heat in microwave for 30 seconds, then mix together thoroughly.

When chicken is almost cooked, add bell peppers and peanut sauce. Mix together thoroughly and cook for 3 minutes. Add bean sprouts and continue to cook for 2 minutes or until chicken is no longer pink inside. Serve on rice vermicelli.

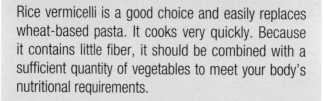

DIGESTIVE HEALTH INFO

• •

Rice vermicelli is a good choice and easily replaces wheat-based pasta. It cooks very quickly. Because it contains little fiber, it should be combined with a sufficient quantity of vegetables to meet your body's nutritional requirements.

Nutrition Facts Per serving	
Amount	
Calories	536
Fat	25 g
Sodium	417 mg
Carbohydrates	43 g
Fiber	5 g
Protein	39 g

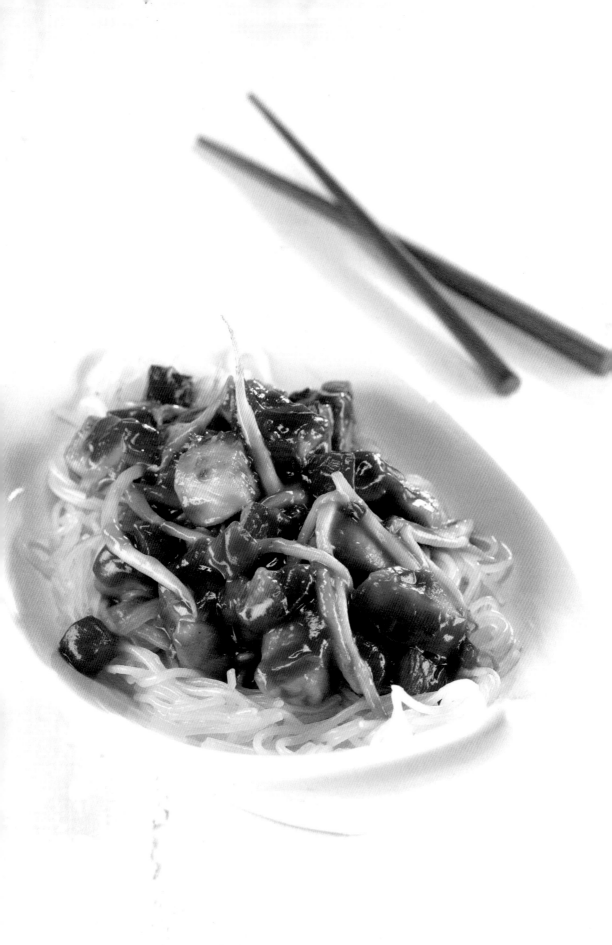

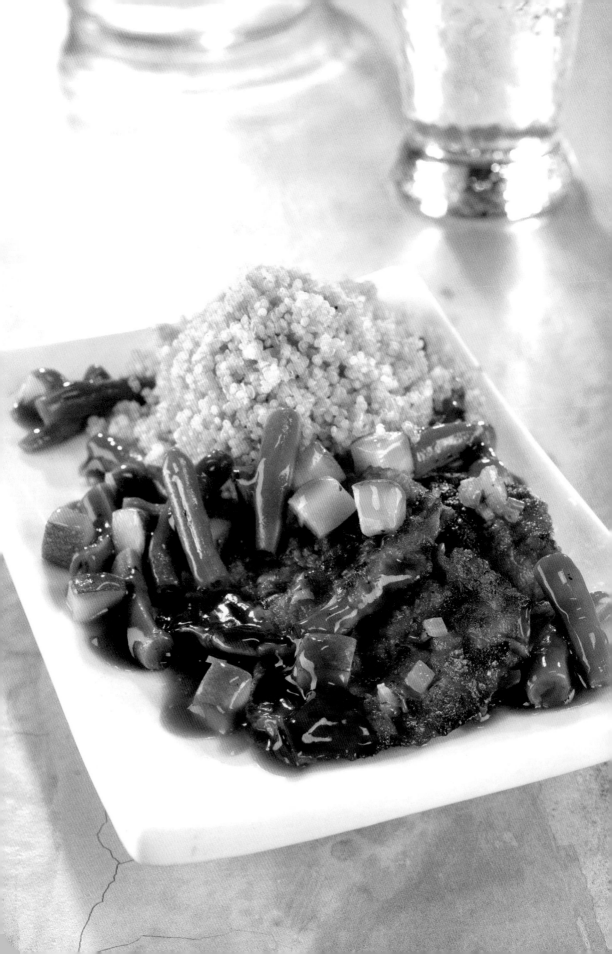

with Vegetables

4 servings • PREPARATION: 30 minutes • COOKING TIME: 20 minutes

METHOD

In a saucepan, combine quinoa and 2 cups (500 ml) water. Bring to a boil and cook for 20 minutes.

Meanwhile, coat slices of beef in cornstarch.

In a skillet, heat oil over medium heat. Add celery and gently fry for 1 to 2 minutes. Add slices of beef and brown for 5 minutes.

Add seasonings, green beans, zucchini and beef broth. Cook over medium-high heat for 3 to 4 minutes until sauce has thickened.

Serve beef with quinoa.

INGREDIENTS

1 cup (250 ml) white quinoa, rinsed and drained

14 oz (390 g) beef, thinly sliced

1 tbsp cornstarch

2 tbsp canola oil

2 stalks celery, chopped

2 cups (500 ml) green beans, cut in pieces

1 zucchini, diced

1 cup (250 ml) low-sodium beef broth

For the seasonings

1 tbsp chopped fresh chive

1 tbsp dried basil

Salt and black pepper

Nutrition Facts
Per serving

Amount	
Calories	415
Fat	14 g
Sodium	800 mg
Carbohydrates	56 g
Fiber	7 g
Protein	33 g

LINGUINI
with Olives

6 servings • PREPARATION: 20 minutes • COOKING TIME: 20 minutes

INGREDIENTS

10 oz (300 g) gluten-free linguini

1 tbsp olive oil

2 stalks celery, chopped

2 cups (500 ml) pitted sliced black olives

½ cup (125 ml) low-sodium chicken broth

2 tbsp gluten-free flour

2 cups (500 ml) lactose-free milk

1 cup (250 ml) chopped ham

4 cups (1 liter) baby spinach leaves

For the seasonings

1 tsp dried thyme

1 tbsp fresh or dried parsley

Salt and black pepper

METHOD

In a large saucepan of boiling water, cook pasta according to directions on package.

In a large skillet, heat oil over medium heat. Add celery and gently fry for 2 to 3 minutes. Add olives, chicken broth and thyme. Continue to cook for 5 minutes.

In a bowl, combine flour and milk. Gradually pour mixture into saucepan. Cook, stirring frequently, for 10 minutes until sauce thickens.

Add ham, parsley, salt and black pepper. Add spinach and cook for 2 to 3 minutes until spinach is wilted.

Mix sauce into pasta.

Nutrition Facts
Per serving

Amount	
Calories	389
Fat	16 g
Sodium	939 mg
Carbohydrates	48 g
Fiber	6 g
Protein	17 g

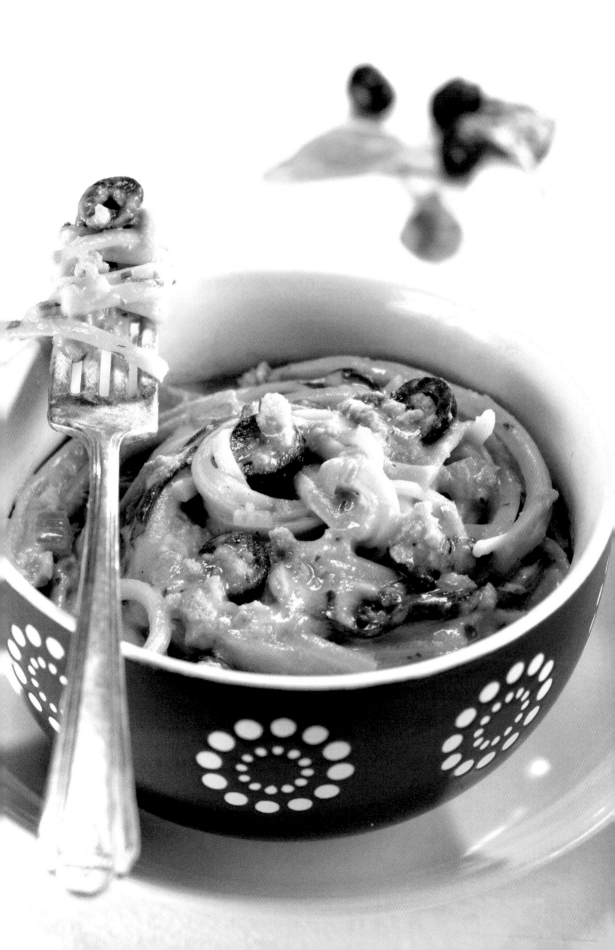

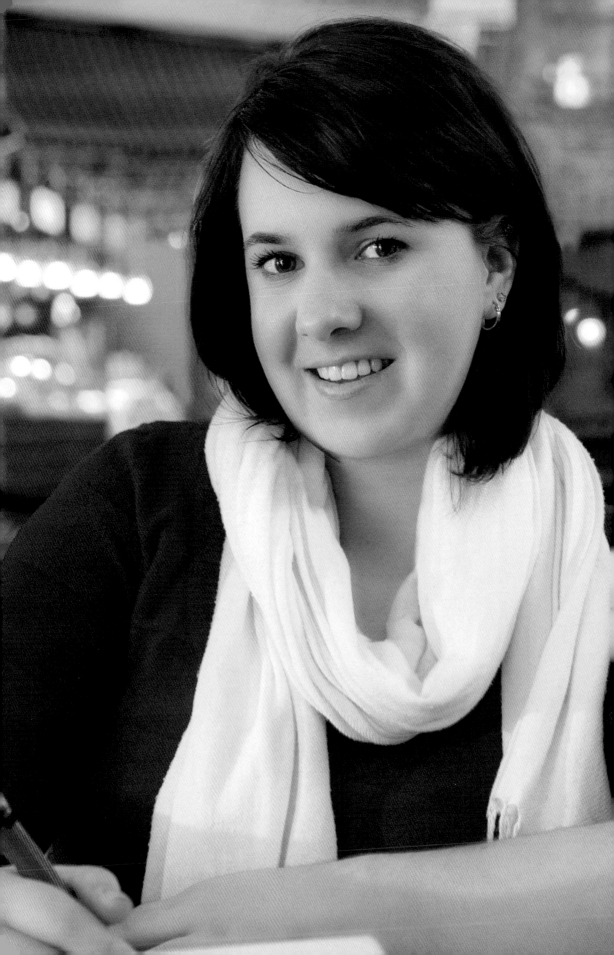

ABOUT
the Author

Alexandra Leduc is a registered dietitian, who graduated in biochemistry and nutrition from Laval University. She is the author of many cookbooks.

She is also the founder of Alex Cuisine (alexcuisine.com), a company that promotes health through healthy and fast cooking. In her classes, which include parent and child coaching and online videos, she presents simple approaches to everyday cooking.

What she loves most is creating delicious recipes with readily available ingredients. "You don't need to raid an organic food store or be a great chef to eat properly," she believes. Alexandra advocates an approach to cooking that is grounded in reality and is a long way from culinary competitions.

She also offers expertise in weight management and helps people develop a healthy relationship with food and achieve a balanced weight, while avoiding diets and restrictions. She has developed an approach — mindful eating — along with an online program (alimentationconsciente.com), which presents tools for applying it daily.

In 2011, she was named Young Business Personality in the professional services category by the Jeune chambre de commerce de Québec (Young Chamber of Commerce of Quebec). In May 2013, she received the Young Woman of the Year award as part of the YWCA Quebec's Women of Distinction gala, and in 2014, Laval University's Alumni Association named her Influential Alumnus.

alexcuisine.com

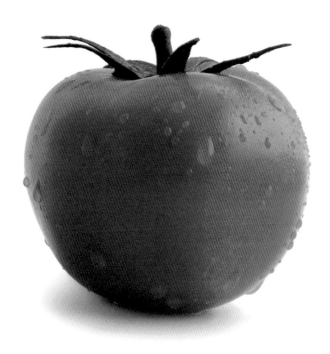

ACKNOWLEDGMENTS

A special thanks to my family and my husband Jean-Philippe. I would surely not have accomplished this without you. Your unconditional support and encouragement make all the difference. Thanks to my mother, Christiane, who cheerfully tests and takes part in making these recipes. Your help is always so precious to me.

Thanks to my friend, nutritionist Laurie Parent-Drolet. Many thanks as well to nutritionist Marie-Pier Tremblay, and to my sister Gabrielle for graciously taking the time to test my recipes.

A special thanks to Groupe Modus, Marc G. Alain and Isabelle Jodoin for your trust and for the great projects you allow me to be part of; you make it such a rewarding experience. Thanks for helping people eat better. Thanks as well to content editor Nolwenn Gouezel for her tips and suggestions, and graphic designers Émilie Houle and Gabrielle Lecompte for the beautiful layout.

I must also mention the work of photographer André Noël, whose magnificent photos always manage to whet the appetite. After all, we eat with our eyes first!

RESOURCES
for Irritable Bowel Syndrome Sufferers

Canadian Digestive Help Foundation
www.cdhf.ca/en/disorders/details/id/12

Irritable Bowel Syndrome Self Help and Support Group
www.ibsgroup.org

The John Hopkins Division of Gastroenterology and Hepatology
www.hopkinsmedicine.org/gastroenterology_hepatology

**International Foundation for Functional Gastrointestinal Disorders
About Irritable Bowel Syndrome**
www.aboutibs.org

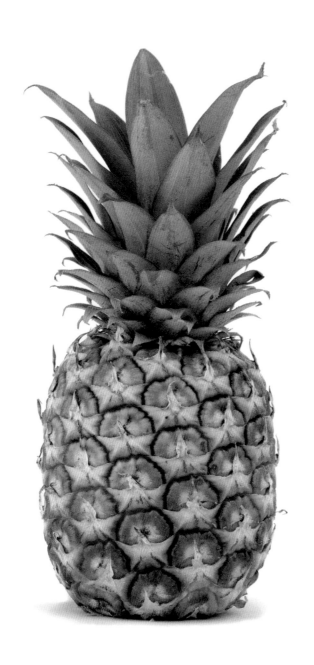

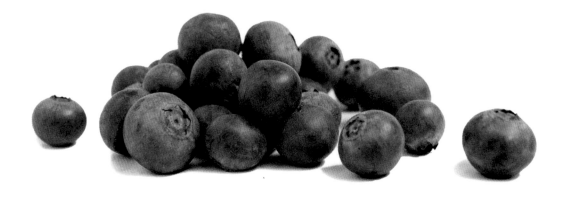

RECIPE
Index

KNOW WHAT TO EAT

A diet suited to your needs based on advice
from **expert dietitians**

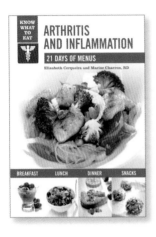

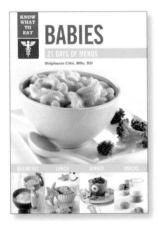

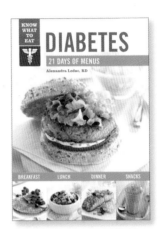

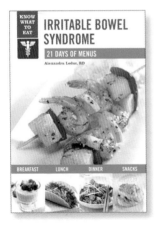

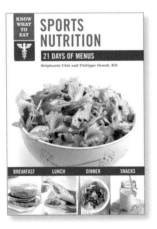

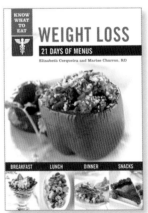

MODUSVIVENDIPUBLISHING.COM